"As the Health and Fitne[   ]ss of over 700 members of our [   ]ubt the information in Patri [   ]k is priceless to anyone looking to obtain optimum health and fitness and to become free from pain-the right way. You will not be disappointed with what this book has to offer."

~Patrick G, Health and Fitness Manager

"Symmetry is what I needed to prepare for my return to competitive mountain bike racing. If you need an overhaul on your body to rid yourself of your chronic issues, then this book is a must read!"

~Mark Shaw, CEO, Total Body Fitness

"I have been using Symmetry's method for 7 years now. It is imperative that you read this book. The information you will receive is life changing!"

~Max "Pain" Griffin, UFC Fighter, West Coast Fighting Champion

"This book will give you the understanding and tools that you need to take control of musculoskeletal pain. Practicing movements that restore normal posture and alignment, and regaining full range of motion in the spine, arms, and legs is a formula for success."

~Stephen Newman, MD

"The Symmetry program is incredible; I've seen it time and again in my clients and have experienced it personally. If you want to get out of pain and build a solid foundation from which your body can thrive, this book is the best place to start!"

~Amy Camacho, Owner, Kaia FIT

"As the owner and head coach of Rock Steady Boxing Warrior Fit, I am devoted to and fiercely protective of my boxers, all of whom have Parkinson's. I can say without reservation or fear of hyperbole

that the results some of my boxers have received through working with Patrick and his wonderful team, are nothing short of miraculous. Do yourself a great favor and read this book!"

~Kevin Quinn, Owner, Rock Steady Boxing

"As an Integrative and Functional Medicine physician, my intention with patients is to address "root causes" of illness rather than just treating symptoms. This book does a fantastic job of explaining the "whys" behind your pain and empowering you to take the needed steps to achieve long term healing. It worked for me, as well as a number of my patients, and it can work for you too!"

~Maxine Barish-Wreden, MD, ABIHM

"As an Integrative Medicine practitioner for over 30 years, I am aware of the importance postural alignment is in overall health and wellness. Patrick has created a system that is highly effective in addressing structural issues and guiding individuals toward healing, and this book provides you the map to understanding the real explanation behind chronic pain."

~Janet M Bailey, PhD

THE PHYSICS OF PAIN

Becoming Pain Free

2nd Edition

PATRICK R. MUMMY

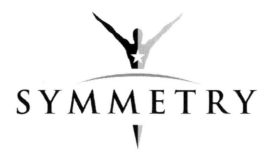

SYMMETRY

DEDICATION

It means everything to me to recognize the people who have stayed the course believing in me and in what I have created. Without each of them, the journey would have been vastly different, to say the least. Following is a short but inspired thank you!

My late wife Lauren was inspiration personified. Her talent as a writer, storyteller, motivator, mother, friend, business partner, and wife, was as good as it gets. I remember her waking up next to me one morning in 2002; she looked at me and said, "You can create something huge with this business, darling. All you have to do is write it down, and you will succeed". I did, and I have. Even during that fateful trip she took to South Africa, she was creating bigger plans for us upon her return. She will always be remembered, honored, and terribly missed.

My daughters Ryenne and Jaide both mean everything to me. They inspire me to be the best I can be, and I am blessed and so grateful to be their father and to see them become the beautiful, intelligent young women they are. Their mother would have been beyond proud.

To my business partners and best friends, both former and present. I met Michael Donnelly, who was my first investor, as a client. When he was 19, he broke his neck cliff-diving off Sunset Cliffs in San Diego. He proved the doctors wrong four-months later by walking again. I met him 26 years later when his injury had started to take its toll. He made such great progress with Symmetry that he invested in my first software program.

Andrew Duenas, a retired Air Force Chief Master Sergeant, had everything in life to pursue after he retired but he chose to join Symmetry and share his vast expertise and knowledge with us. His unwavering support to our cause has been nothing short of heroic.

Adam Frick, the first and only programmer to create the software I can stand behind.

I fixed Andy Rocklin's knee. He fixed my life. I have never in my short time on this planet met someone as humble as he is, as willing to jump in at a moment's notice, give advice if asked, and never complain about his return on investment, or lack thereof! The man is patient, and without him, this book would not have been written.

Finally, Lee Anne. I never really knew what unconditional love meant until I met her. Her passion and unrelenting support of me, my family, and my business, are a huge reason for my personal and business success. There are certain people in our chapters of life that if we had not met, would have changed the course of our future. I love this woman and will never take this gift for granted.

What I love about the 25 years of being in this field, is meeting people that I can honestly call great friends and mentors. I have evaluated nearly 10,000 people in my career, including: Az Hakim who I watched play at San Diego State and win a Super Bowl as a Ram; Tony Gwynn, who flew me out to Peoria, AZ during Spring Training; and, Steve Emtman who forced me to train him in Symmetry when I still didn't have a clue what I was doing. To people like Bill Randoll who has never stopped believing in me; and to all the clients who have come into Symmetry, willing to change their lives and take control of their health. These and all my clients are the people I dedicate this book to because not only have I been able to get to know these people intimately but changing a paradigm does not come just from a method. It comes from relationships and having those who believe in you enough to help penetrate and change the establishment.

~Patrick Mummy

CONTENTS

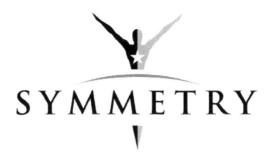

SYMMETRY

FOREWORD

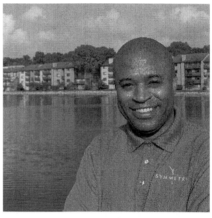

I want to let as many people know about Symmetry as possible, although many people are slow to warm up to new ideas when they do not know enough about something to truly value it. I know Symmetry changes lives because it changed mine. I also know, once people witness through their own experience how incredibly effective this technology is, they will value it indefinitely.

Patrick Mummy and I met back in 2005 when I was working with a trainer and former National Football League (NFL) player and coach, named Harland Svare. During the off-season, Harland worked to prepare me for the rigorous battles of the NFL. One day while training with several partners who were already battling injuries, a friend of mine began experiencing back issues that prevented him from working out. Harland, seeing my partner injured and in pain, decided to schedule an appointment to take us to Patrick's office in La Jolla. We did not even practice that morning; we just went straight to his office.

When I introduced myself, Patrick's eyes lit up! As it turned out, he had been a fan of mine for quite some time. He followed my career from the time I played at his Alma Mater, San Diego State University,

1

until I played for the St. Louis Rams and won a Super Bowl championship in 2000. We had parallel lives but never connected until that day.

From the very beginning, Patrick and I hit it off. He told me about his company and what it was about and assured me that if I ever needed him, he would be there for me. I knew immediately that he was a man of his word and I could rely on him. Looking back now, I should have taken the initiative right there on the spot to go through a routine. I was not necessarily hurting at the time—and did not understand that this technology would help me even though I was not hurting. I was not able to fully reap the benefits of Symmetry during our first introduction.

In 2005, I went to a training camp with the New Orleans Saints. It was the year of Hurricane Katrina, so our training took place in San Antonio, Texas. At practice, I broke a tackle and immediately tried to accelerate after spinning off a teammate. Being that my body was not in alignment, and because of my attempt to accelerate from the misaligned position I was in, I pulled my hamstring. I was out for six weeks before I was even able to participate and practice fully with my teammates. I knew I had to do something. Even more, I knew that the traditional methods of help were not doing enough to get me up to speed and back in the game. I would get a treatment and be asked how I was feeling each time, then be sent out prematurely only to reinjure my hamstring. This happened to me three times before I realized what I was missing. I called Patrick and flew him out to San Antonio. Once we were together, Patrick immediately took my measurements. He told me one hip was elevated six degrees higher than the other and rotated forward, and then explained this was the main reason I was experiencing problems. I was astounded. I laughed at him. "Yeah, go figure!" I said. However, after taking my measurements, Patrick then created and took me through my first sequence of corrective exercises.

After leading me through my routine he asked me to walk and then jog. I didn't feel any hamstring tightness or tension in my long gate. I was amazed at the benefits I immediately received from his treatment. I was impressed. I was on the field the next day practicing with my

2

teammates, and I never struggled with my hamstring again. Experiencing the restoration of my abilities after not being able to train a single day for the previous six weeks made me realize his technology was a game-changer. In that moment, I became an official believer in Patrick and in Symmetry.

Integrating Symmetry's Postural Alignment Technology™ into my daily routine did tremendous wonders for my being—both my body and soul. I was able to think more clearly. Through the process of realigning my body, something amazing happened. It seemed my use of the technology not only aligned my body but prepared me mentally for each day. For the first time, I felt aligned physically and spiritually. I noticed I was able to focus longer, think more clearly, push myself physically without fear of injury, and I no longer experienced kinks in my neck that I periodically had after a night of sleeping crookedly. Most days, after completing my routine, I discovered the remainder of my day flowed in such a way that I was able to achieve whatever I had set out for the day. I was determined to continue my routine throughout (and beyond) the rest of my NFL career. It has helped me tremendously both professionally and personally. This program, in many ways, changed my life.

I was not the only one to experience these incredible results. My family went through Symmetry as well. My father, who struggled with back issues and lethargy was able to alleviate his back pain altogether while simultaneously increasing his energy levels. All while the doctors continued to recommend surgery. My teammates noticed a shift too. While I was going through Symmetry, Patrick was also working with a few of my teammates, Ernie Conwell, and Steve Gleason to name a couple. These guys were very invested in taking care of their bodies. They knew Patrick was on to something when he worked with them and their alignment. It takes extreme skill to know what is wrong with your body, how to identify the problem, and then to take an isometric exercise and use it to rebuild your body. This knowledge was key to us.

One day while Patrick and I were meeting he mentioned one of my teammates to me, Deuce McAllister. Patrick told me, quite vehemently, that he wanted me to speak to Deuce on his behalf and asked me to bring him into the clinic. Patrick believed he was favoring his left leg and was vulnerable to a right knee injury because of it. I found this assessment odd because I knew Deuce did not have any knee or leg problems at the time. Regardless, Patrick believed Deuce was on the verge of a serious injury due to how severely he was compensating with his right leg, and he believed his program could help if he were given the chance to meet with him.

Two weeks later Patrick came to visit me to see how my body was responding to the corrective routine. When I saw him, I immediately asked him how he could have possibly predicted Deuce's knee injury. Patrick had not even known, but in-between trips, Deuce had suffered a severe right-knee injury, an injury that he incurred without ever coming into direct contact with another player. And Patrick said it was going to happen! It was an unfortunate accident that Patrick had been trying to get Deuce to avoid, though he never got the opportunity.

An incredible toll is placed on your body when you play a high-performance sport competitively, and athletes need to understand there is life after sports. Symmetry is designed to help at any stage of a competitive athletic career: before, during, and after. The reality, however, is that so many people wait until they are in pain to do something about it. What most people do not realize is the empowerment in and importance of taking preventative measures to ensure your body stays healthy in all circumstances.

An even bigger reality, which is the reason Postural Alignment Technology™ is having such a difficult time breaking into the professional sports arena, is that people fear change. In other words, what is new and what they do not know. Quite frankly, implementing Symmetry's Postural Alignment Technology™ into sports medicine would leave a lot of people without jobs. The trainers who assess sports injury rely heavily on players to continue getting injured to maintain job security. It is an ugly truth that needs to be stated. For example, if injuries were being addressed at the cause, rather than after the effect,

4

many sports medicine trainers would be out of a job. Instead, these trainers and people in high-powered positions continue handing athlete's old remedies like "ice and stim", and "rest is best". However, if your body is not in proper alignment then the treatment you receive never has the chance to address the root of the problem, and therefore your body is never able to fully recover. This explains why so many athletes become injured, go through typical treatment protocols, recuperate, are injured shortly after recuperating, and the cycle continues. The effect, rather than the cause of pain, is being treated. Symmetry is the first method I know of that does not treat symptoms; it addresses the cause of pain, removing the symptoms altogether.

It is extremely important for high performance businesses, with athletes playing at the highest levels, and where competitive sports place a great demand on an athlete's body, to find a form of treatment that works—particularly where professional athletes are concerned. Instead, injury is the new lifestyle. People would rather wake up and ice an ankle than wake up with a routine, simply because it is what they are used to doing. Nevertheless, if you are not waking up with a routine, and actively seeking to get your body in proper alignment, your body's compensation patterns will eventually wear you down. This will cause an injury to arise again and again regardless of whether you are a professional athlete, or not.

My hope is to communicate to all higher-ups, both in professional sports and healthcare, that Symmetry defines the new format of training and performance. Bringing your body into proper and maximized alignment is the most efficient and effective way for one to take their performance to the next level. When a person aligns their body, they are better equipped and able to focus on a rigorous workout. It is because of this that Symmetry belongs in every sport, in every college program, in every gym, sports medicine and physical therapy book, and certainly in every home: if you're playing a sport, Symmetry needs to be implemented into your daily routine; if you are a coach, your players need to have these routines; if you maintain a sports medicine or physical therapy program for your athletes or patients, it needs to utilize Symmetry. Symmetry's Postural Alignment Technology protects the body from the inside out and preserves the longevity of a person's physical abilities. Every person interested in taking care of their body needs to invest in a routine. You need to take care of your body and it will take care of you. It works if you work it!

I thank Patrick. He is my brother from another mother. He is also on this planet to help people, serve people, and make a difference in this world. Patrick means the world to me because he has done an incredible amount for me. Without him, Symmetry would not have been created, and it is his creation of the Symmetry Technology that has given me the light to progress further in life. I know what it did for me, and I am confident that it can change someone else's life the way it has changed mine.

The book you are about to read will change you; whether you are a practitioner who wants to enhance your practice, or someone in need of a solution to your chronic pain. It is a beautiful combination of Patrick's personal journey in creating Symmetry, to the technical understanding of how Symmetry works. My greatest aspiration is that through careful study of the Symmetry method, you will be empowered, and with Patrick's guidance and direction, alleviate your pain and improve your health.

~Az Hakim

SAN DIEGO STATE UNIVERSITY 1992

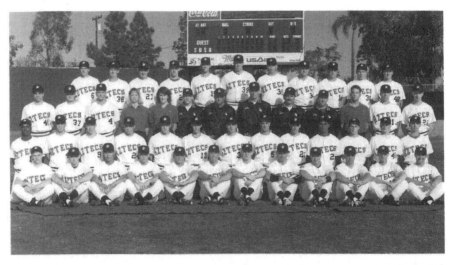

Front row: (l-r) Jim Judevine, Pat Mummy, Tony Enomoto, Keith Tripp, Terry Picchiottino, Jason Ledford, Dan Drewien, Marcelino Garcia, Rick Page, Rick Navarro, Steve Dietz, Mark Papadopoulos. Second row: Tony Robertson, Steve Trainor, Matt Cleek, Brad Gennaro, Ryan Nettles, John Lynn, Benji Grigsby, Beau Champoux, Richie Juarez, Malcolm Warfield, Jim Rushford, Greg Quam, Brent Ferguson. Third row: Mike Kendall, Walt Bills, Ryan Bills, Brenda Czaplinski (Trainer), Adrienne Wassel (Trainer), Matt DeSales, Jim Dietz (Head Coach), Matt Haar (Asst. Coach), Pat Oliverio (Asst. Coach), Jim Warner (Asst. Coach), Will Laskey (Trainer), Clint Borman, Derek Vinyard. Fourth row: Matt Franco, Brian Kochner, James Davis, Jerry Stafford, Craig Kenney, Mike Barber, Scott Hofstede, Mark Gapski, Jay Hassel, Doug Webb, Rob Callaway.

"I was stretched, pulled, kneaded, taped, injected, iced, and adjusted, only to get temporary relief at best."

~ Patrick Mummy

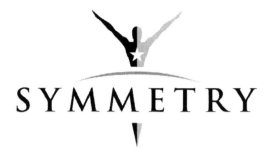

SYMMETRY

RELIANCE

It was the top of the ninth, two outs, the last game of the year, the last play of my career. We were playing the Rainbow Warriors of Hawaii and we desperately wanted to win our last game in what culminated in the strangest season I have ever experienced. The batter hit a ground ball up the middle and as I chased it into center field, I planted my left foot to make the play only to have my ankle give way, again. Instantly, just like that, my career was over.

I had earned a scholarship to San Diego State University (SDSU), a Division One National Collegiate Athletic Association (NCAA) school. Having come from a town of only 1000 people, this was a big deal. I had always wanted to play on a Division One team and through hard work and determination I had achieved that goal. Baseball to me was my priority and college was just the avenue by which I could obtain that goal. The irony was that my chronic injuries brought me knowledge that I was not exactly searching for at the time—a full understanding of the limitations and ineffectiveness of our healthcare system. I chose SDSU for two reasons: 1) it didn't snow there, and 2) it was the only college that offered me a scholarship that had anything related to Physical Therapy, the career I once thought I wanted to pursue when my baseball career was over.

I knew that I wanted to be in a field where I could help people in some way, but no colleges with Physical Therapy and baseball ever recruited me. So, when it came down to choosing from the four schools that did offer me scholarships, I chose SDSU because at that time their Athletic Training program was number two in the nation and offered a natural stepping stone to Physical Therapy school once I graduated. What I did not anticipate was that choosing the combination of Athletic Training and baseball would change my life forever.

I entered my senior year still carrying the dream of becoming a professional major leaguer. I grew up listening to Vin Scully on the radio, spending every opportunity I could listening to the Dodgers over the waves, envisioning myself as Steve Sax turning double plays or leading off in game one of the World Series. It was the one thing I was passionate about as a boy, and then a young man, and I was so close to making it a reality. So, it was natural for me to take the summer and fall going into my final season more seriously than ever before, preparing myself mentally and physically beyond anything I had done in the past. I thought I had the inside track to becoming more physically fit and knowledgeable than I had ever been by being in the Athletic Training program. I lived in the weight room and studied harder than I had ever before.

I went from bench pressing 200 pounds at the end of my junior year, to 300 pounds at the beginning of my senior year. I also earned the Western Athletic Scholar Athlete of the Year award that year. However, I was also chronically injured, worse than ever before, and no one could help me. It was an incredibly frustrating experience to train day and night, yet still have to see every practitioner I could from physical therapists to chiropractors to the team physician. I was stretched, pulled, kneaded, taped, injected, iced, and adjusted, only to get temporary relief at best. This was not supposed to happen. I was in a field that was supposed to provide the answers for injury and pain, but no one could give me the answers I was looking for to heal my pain. Chronic ankle sprains, foot pain, left hamstring pulls, right Sacral Iliac pain, knee and shoulder pain. It was a season of cyclic annoyances that ultimately led me to question the choice of career I had been pursuing.

After I had sprained my ankle in that last game, I was devastated. Despite all my injuries, my determination to play kept me off the bench until that last game. I was voted Most Valuable Player for our team and an All Western Player in the Western Athletic Conference. I was even invited to try out with the St. Louis Cardinals who came to our campus a week later to give us a shot at the next level. Sadly, I could not walk, let alone run or pivot. During the week prior to the tryout, I rehabbed my ankle just as I had so many times before, but on the day of the tryout I showed up to the training room to get taped, and it was locked. Being the end of May, the semester was over and therefore no need to keep the training room open. I stared through the window in front of the training room for about 30-minutes, hoping someone would show up to tape me. This was where I had my first revelation. I realized for the first time how dependent I was on practitioners fixing me when I had an injury, and the moment when I needed one the most, I found myself alone and helpless—I panicked.

The St. Louis Cardinals was a dream opportunity. My sister had bought me a miniature St. Louis Cardinals bat 15 years prior when she went on a trip to Missouri. I was sure that by holding onto that bat all those years I'd secured my fate, and now I'd been invited to try out for them. However, I found myself hopeless on the most important day of my life up to that point, all the years of hard work and determination were seemingly for naught. This was not how my career was supposed to end. In fact, I never really planned for it to end. Nonetheless, I knew that on that particular day, due to our team's disastrous record of 22 wins and 44 losses that season, not many scouts had showed up to observe our players and this would probably be my one shot to make it to the next level. Yet, here I stood, helpless and feeling sorry for myself, and ready to give up. Somehow, I pulled myself together, went home to my apartment, and taped my own ankle.

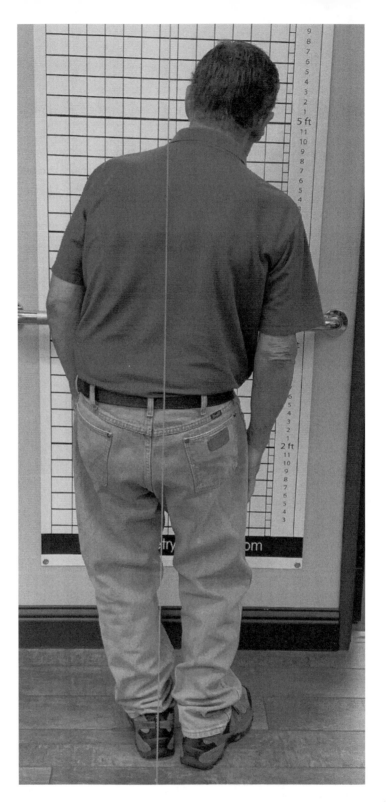

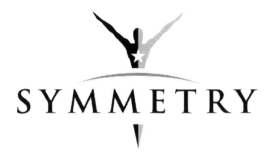

SYMMETRY

POSTURE AND PAIN

There are no coincidences in life, in my opinion. After realizing that my career path needed to change, one day while running on the beach I literally ran into a former classmate. She was a great friend who I often studied and hung out with, and after apologizing for colliding into her, I explained why I was in such deep thought, unaware that she was in my path. After listening to my woes about not knowing what career to choose, she smiled and excitedly told me the clinic she worked for was looking to hire, and what they specialized in was not taught in school, nor were they looking for anyone with great experience. I immediately went home, called the clinic, applied, and was offered a position the following week! In one instant my life had changed. It felt good to have direction again.

The interview process was a bit backwards. Typically, I would be meeting first with the head of the Athletic Program, Harland Svare, the former New York Giant who was in charge of the athletic program. Then I was to meet with the director of therapy, and after that, the founder of the Egoscue Method itself, Pete Egoscue. However, I met first with Pete because the director and Harland were away on business. Pete is a large barrel-chested man with the bed-side manner of a retired marine (he is a retired marine). When I met with him, he was silent at first, intimidatingly so, while observing me walk into the clinic. I shook his hand and we walked to his office.

Once inside, Pete began by asking me if I had ever heard of him or his clinic before, and I explained that I had not. He then asked me why I applied for this job. I filled him in about my past and explained my disappointment in the western medical model. I told him that I was looking for a program that I could believe in and that could possibly help me with my injuries. He laughed and said, "If you end up working here, and with what you will be learning, you really should be paying us!" I did not know how to take that as I had no idea what he had created, but he started to explain. What he explained blew me away.

Upon observing me and knowing I had played baseball, Pete told me exactly how I stood in the batter's box, where I tended to hit the ball, and where I more than likely had my pain. He had nailed it right on the spot. I was really impressed. He was too. But I gave him latitude as no one had ever assessed me in a way that did not involve x-rays and stethoscopes or muscle testing. I finally knew I had found my calling.

For the next two weeks I dedicated my time to studying the roughly 300 stretches and isometric strengthening positions. Some I had learned in college, others were offshoots of yoga poses, and some I had never seen before. After that, my training consisted of observing the therapists, asking as many questions as I could, and trying to figure out how this method worked. Two months later, I showed up to work one day and they had overbooked their clients. I was given my first client to take through on my own; thus, began my career as a Postural Therapist. I had no idea what I was doing.

There was no test for me to take, no observation of me proving I knew what I was doing. There were no manuals for me to reference. There were no steps for me to follow in creating a menu for my clients. However, I knew the philosophy was sound. If you have poor posture you are compromising your joints when you move, which can cause pain. The problem I had was that the entire method was based on viewing a person's posture and watching them walk. The process was extremely subjective, and it was hard to prove what changes had been made from session to session, especially if the client was not getting out of pain. Most clients did eventually get better going through the program, but only after great cost and time.

Not only was this method expensive, but the time it took to go through the sequence of exercises was on average 60 minutes per attempt. Why? Because there was no quantification of the method. Clients had to strip down to their underwear for us to observe their asymmetries. Then, as if that wasn't uncomfortable enough, we would take their pictures. . Our only reference point for the success of the program was the pain itself. This was no different than any other treatment I had experienced. Even the most committed client would eventually stop doing their routine because it took too much time. Unfortunately, and since our ability to create routines was so subjective, we would end up giving too many exercises just hoping that something would stick.

I knew I was in the right field, but I also knew I was running out of passion working at this clinic. The reason I pressed on was because the method worked for me when everything else had not. Two years later I realized it was time to go out on my own. I wanted to develop a better system that was capable of yielding results based on a quantifiable measurement process.

I remember the exact day I made the decision to leave. I was working with a client who I had never seen before but was still experiencing a lot of pain after five sessions, and I had no idea what to do with her. I elicited the help of the director. He came out, firmly gazed at my client as she walked up and down the hall, suggested a series of stretches, and walked away. I went to my office to digest his list and began pulling my hair out as I had no clue why he sequenced these exercises in the order he had chosen. With a frustrated sigh, I decided to elicit the guidance of Pete Egoscue. Pete always stood with his arms folded and one hand caressing his chin while in deep thought. After my client walked back and forth several times, Pete turned to me and commanded his orders. I quickly receded back to my office to digest his menu of exercises.

That was when I confirmed my second revelation. The two recommended sequences of exercises for the client were not at all the same. At that moment I realized that instinct alone cannot be taught. Also, this process needed consistency and standardization to fully be considered a method. The next day Symmetry was born, and I have never looked back.

I formally started Symmetry in 1997 with the assumption that I knew how to run a business. I was 27 and ignorant. Coupled with starting a business, I had married as well. I honestly believe that if everyone knew what it took to create a successful business, and marriage, for that matter, not many businesses (or marriages) would exist. I suppose that is why more businesses and marriages fail than succeed.

I had taken what I had learned at the Egoscue Method and simply applied it to the new business, still not really knowing what I was doing, but understanding enough to get people out of pain. I knew in my heart that this was not good enough. Apparently, I had sent out that message because it was not too long after that I received a phone call from a man named Geoff Gluckman. Geoff had also worked for Egoscue and left to start his own company a few years previous. He asked me if I was confident in what I had learned. Of course, he knew what my answer would be and so instead I asked him what was different with his method. The conversation piqued my attention enough to sign up for his course, as I had so desperately wanted some type of education while working at the Egoscue clinic. Geoff provided me with the next revelation by reintroducing me to the planes of motion. I had studied the planes of motion in college for about a day. The planes of motion are the ways the body moves around gravity and give a basis for how the body operates three-dimensionally. Geoff had put Egoscue's ideas into a concrete way of explaining how the body works around right angles. His method provided a baseline of understanding how asymmetries are derived, and therefore how to correct them.

This, however, only went so far. I still found myself not fully understanding the process of sequencing, even though the planes of motion concept at least gave me some indication of how to compare and compartmentalize the deviations I was seeing. I vividly remember a heated debate between a chiropractor and Geoff at his Level 3 course. There was great confusion about why Geoff picked a certain exercise in one of his examples, and why it was a better choice for the particular deviation he was discussing. The argument went on for about 30 minutes and the chiropractor could not get Geoff to explain his theory well enough for him to let it go, and in the end, Geoff told him to just trust his explanation. Deja vu. I had heard that phrase about 50 times while working at the Egoscue clinic, and I realized at that moment that there had to be a better way to explain this system beyond Geoff's theory. It was good, but not great. I found myself still at a loss of explanations that satiated my desire to fully understand how this therapy worked. I began to search more.

Two weeks later, I was speaking to one of my clients about my experience with Gluckman, and they mentioned a chiropractor in Newport Beach that they knew who thought outside the box. I really do not know what prompted me to contact this doctor, but the timing seemed appropriate, so I called. He was a nice older gentleman who specialized in Atlas Orthogonal work; fine neck adjustments to clear the nerve pathways from the base of the head to the body. What impressed me the most though was all the gadgets he had in his office to show his patients how misaligned they were. He had a glass footplate with a camera underneath to show the pressure imbalances of the feet while standing. He had a force plate analyzer that showed how the weight was divided on both legs. But one gadget impressed me the most—a fancy level that his neighbor had made for him that measured the elevation of the pelvis.

A simple bubble showed his patient how uneven their pelvis was while standing, and then how even the bubble was after making one simple adjustment to the neck. What caught my attention the most wasn't the device itself, but the reaction the patient had once they were re-measured with the level. They were impressed with how the bubble leveled out and how this correlated directly to a decrease in the pain they were experiencing. His patient was giddy with enthusiasm and it was at this moment that I realized the missing link from my experiences with Egoscue and Gluckman. Neither had an objective way of measuring their outcomes; therefore, no way to monitor their progress from session to session. This doctor had positively affected the patient's experience by providing them with a better understanding of why they felt relief. I realized that I had lacked the same experiences in college and that my only reference to the success of a treatment was whether I felt better or not. Unfortunately, for me, I had no long-term relief and no explanations as to why, which is the story I hear every day at my clinic.

I knew in that moment that I had to make one of these devices myself. I asked the chiropractor if his neighbor would make one for me, but he no longer lived near him. I immediately went to Home Depot to try and build one myself but failed miserably. Again, timing.

I was obsessed with the burning idea of figuring out how to take what Gluckman taught me and make it into an objective process. While I was sitting at a warehouse in Oceanside, waiting to pick up Symmetry shirts, I found a device called the Palpation Meter in a medical catalog I was glancing through. It reached out at me like one of those pop-up books I used to read as a kid. I immediately ordered one and thus began the process of Postural Alignment Technology™.

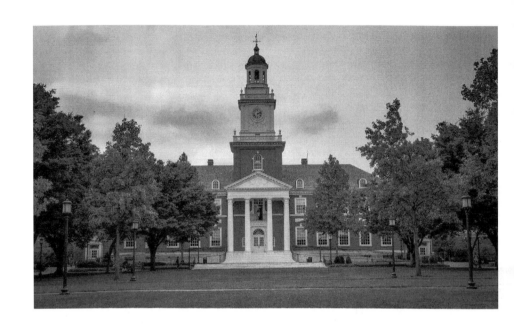

"The annual cost of chronic pain is as high as $635 billion a year, which is more than the yearly costs for cancer, heart disease, and diabetes."

~Health Economists at John Hopkins University

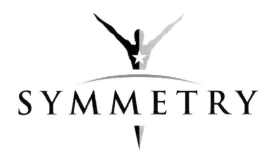

SYMMETRY

UNDERSTANDING PAIN

If there is one thing I would like to disseminate to anyone who is suffering from chronic pain, it is simply to help the person understand WHY he or she is in pain, and how our current medical model is not addressing it correctly. Look at these statistics regarding chronic pain:

- The National Institute of Health reported that low back pain (LBP) is the second most common cause of disability in adults in the United States, and a common reason for lost workdays. An estimated 149 million days of work per year are lost due to LBP.

- Health Economists from Johns Hopkins University reported in *The Journal of Pain*, reported that the annual cost of chronic pain is as high as $635 billion a year, which is more than the yearly costs for cancer, heart disease, and diabetes combined.

- New research by economists in the United States and Iceland, using a massive government survey of Americans over age 50, estimated in a new working paper published by the *National Bureau of Economic Research* (August, 2017) that living with chronic pain makes people so unhappy that they'd need to earn between $20,000 and $50,000 per year more to be as happy as they would be otherwise with no pain. Another way to say it, people would pay between $56 and $145 per day to be just as happy as they are otherwise, but pain-free. (Vox.com)

Being in this field for 25 years now, the one thing that always makes me cringe is that the amount of chronic pain in our society increases each year. With all the technological advancements, the newest surgeries, and the latest drugs, pain and disease become more and more prevalent each year. How can this be with all the brilliant minds in our medical community? To me it is simple. Prevention versus reaction. The emphasis of treatment is completely backwards as we focus almost completely on the pain or disease itself rather than the cause of the pain or disease. Think about it: What are the treatment recommendations for chronic pain? Medication is most prevalent, followed by physical therapy, hands-on treatments, and then surgery if all else fails. The common denominator with all these treatment models is a reliance on something or someone to make you feel better. No one program gives you a comprehensive home plan, with consistent follow-up and adjustments, to make sure you are not only staying consistent with the program, but making the proper changes to allow you to maintain and sustain progress. Most therapies certainly do not focus on preventing the issues from coming back, rather, the focus is on temporary symptom relief.

I was at a health fair once in San Diego, and I was speaking to the CEO of the corporation we were sponsoring. He was from Japan and we were talking about Symmetry because he was intrigued by our concept of prevention to get rid of pain. If you genuinely think about it, almost all disease and pain can be prevented if you are knowledgeable about what it is you are trying to prevent. However, most people do not know what they do not know, and so proceed with the mantra "if it isn't broke, don't fix it". This CEO was explaining that Eastern philosophy is all about prevention.

Most Japanese corporations have their employees perform some type of yoga or stretching before they start their day. Yoga not only helps physically, but it builds morale, thus increasing employee production. He further explained that when something critical does occur, the Japanese come to the United States because we are known for our great reactive medical care. Who do you think is saving the most money overall? I know this is another topic, healthcare, but if you are interested in my opinion, it does not matter what the healthcare system is called, but where the focus should be to help people. Our healthcare system is not focused on helping people get better and stay better.

So, is pain a good thing? No, it is great! A chiropractor once explained pain in a way I had never heard before, and I have never forgotten what he said. He told me that pain and our reaction to it is like the smoke detector in your house. What would happen if one night your alarm went off? What would you do? My first reaction would be to check for a fire. But what happens if there is no fire? This has happened to me. My alarm went off, I checked for a fire, which there was not, but the alarm kept blaring. It was 2:30 in the morning so I did what most people would do—I ripped it out of the ceiling! But what if an hour later I had awoken to a real fire? What most of us do not understand is that once you start to feel chronic pain—it does not matter where it is—your body has been compensating for years to avoid it. However, before we talk comprehensively about compensation, we must first discuss what true alignment looks like and why our bodies become misaligned in the first place.

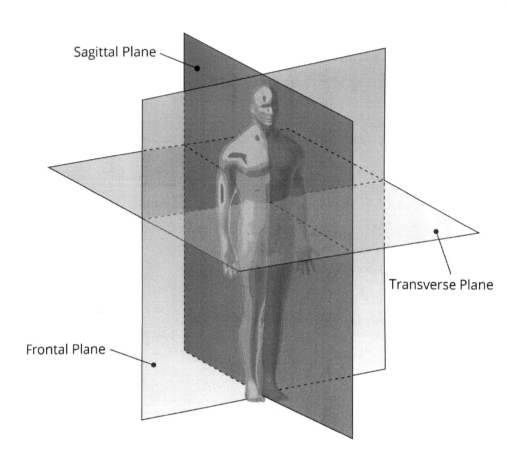

Planes of Motion

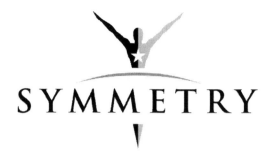

SYMMETRY

TRUE ALIGNMENT

On average, it takes most children 12 months from the time they are born to accomplish their first step. Compared to other mammals, why does it take us so much longer to learn how to walk? Simply put, we are bipedal, or two-legged. In neuromuscular terms, it takes us longer to walk because we evolved to be vertical, and the process of being stable in a vertical position requires a very distinct learning process. We must learn to balance first, then stand, and then walk. The human body has 650 muscles broken into two general types—intrinsic and dynamic. Intrinsic muscles are the core muscles. No, I do not mean abs. Intrinsic muscles are designed to hold your body in a static standing position. Intrinsic muscles do not change length with external force.

Dynamic muscles are the strength muscles. These are designed to move your body. These muscles do change length with external force. When we are learning to walk, we must go through an extremely specific process of educating these two muscle groups to properly work together to efficiently and effectively hold and move our bodies. When we are first born, our initial position is on our backs. Then we learn how to roll ourselves onto our stomachs. Then we crawl. Then we sit. Eventually, we start to pull ourselves up to a standing position, and finally we take our first steps. This process is crucial to the proper development of our body for a plethora of reasons, which we will discuss. But none of it can be understood unless we talk about gravity.

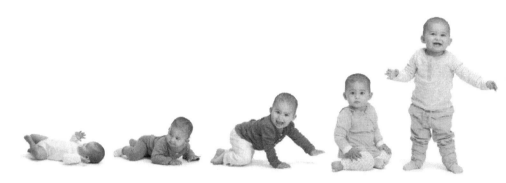

When you have seen your doctor or specialist about your chronic pain, how many of them ever used the word gravity in discussing your issues? No one has ever told me that they discuss gravity with their practitioner. Why not? Because we take it for granted. Right now, you are probably sitting inside of some type of building while you are reading this book. Did you ever once consider whether the building is going to fall on you at any moment? No, because you assumed that the architects who designed it knew what they were doing. What you assumed is that the foundation is level and strong, and that the walls are vertical to the foundation and supporting the ceiling, which is horizontal to the floor. Every day we take things for granted, from the car we drive to the chairs we sit in, assuming they have been built correctly, but never do we consider the force they are constructed around. Understanding the laws of gravity are paramount to understanding the nature of our physical body.

If we were to assess how the human body is designed, how would we conclude the most efficient way for it to operate, both from a physical and physiological perspective? First and foremost, we would know that there is a force that falls perpendicular to the earth's surface through the center of the earth. For the sake of our discussion here, it is not relevant to go deeper into the universal forces and theories, but rather that we all agree that gravity not only exists, but that it is constant. Based on this knowledge, we can take any architectural or engineering principals and apply them to our structure. Let us go back and look at being a child again. Recall that we discussed that it takes an average of one year to stand up straight on our two feet.

During this process, there is a very sequential pattern of development between the brain and the body. Again, for our discussion here, let us not delve into the specifics of neuromuscular makeup. Rather, let us focus on how we would best take a human body and allow it to work the most efficiently around the downward force of gravity. Breaking it down further, we must conclude two things. One, the human body cannot exist without gravity. Two, there must be a universal design that best fits around gravity because this force is constant. The reason it takes one year for us to learn how to walk is because movement is the most important aspect of our function and existence. The brain must coordinate the neurological development between the intrinsic and dynamic muscles around gravity in a way that best supports the entire system.

This is all necessary to maximize movement. When we are born, we do not have the neurological connection to our muscles to allow us to stand and walk immediately. Why is this so important to understand? Once again, I must emphasize that on average it takes us one complete year to be able to walk on two legs. This process of neurological coordination defines how our bodies were meant to be aligned, because once we learn how to move, we do not stop moving, or at least we should not! Given that moving is so crucial to our existence, we must have the form to support the movement properly, thus the phrase "form follows function" was born.

Now that we have established the importance of gravity, let us take a closer look at children once they learn how to move. If you have children or have observed them, you will see that they cannot sit still. This is because the brain is created in such a way that movement feeds its growth and evolution. This is an entire topic in and of itself, but for now, let us stick to the phrase we just mentioned. If movement is priority number one, and form is the mechanism by which we create efficient and effective movement, then we must discuss what true form is, as it relates to the necessity of movement. This is where planes of motion are vital to the overall message of this book, because it defines what true alignment is and should be.

The Planes of Motion was a topic in college that we spent about 20 minutes discussing. I not only have a patent created around these principals, but I have developed a two-year curriculum and intend to make Symmetry an optional Associate of Arts degree.

We currently have a five-level certification program for practitioners, empowering them to apply these principles directly within their practices. So, what are these "Planes of Motion" that are so central to my mission? We mentioned earlier about intrinsic and dynamic muscles. As a reminder, intrinsic muscles hold posture and dynamic muscles enable movement.

| Frontal | Sagittal | Transverse |

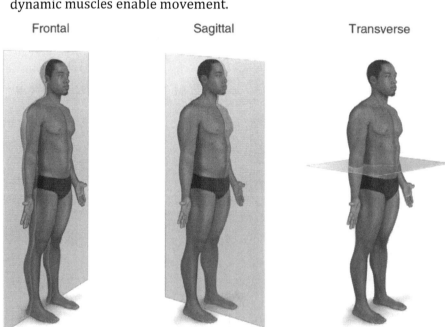

The above diagram shows us is not only proper alignment, but the proper starting position by which the body can move three-

28

dimensionally as efficiently as possible. We can either move side to side (abduction/adduction), which is known as the Coronal Plane or the **Frontal Plane**, front to back (flexion/extension), which is known as the **Sagittal Plane**, or twist (rotation), which is known as the **Transverse Plane**. This alignment is what children show us. From the side view (Frontal Plane) gravity should directly fall through the midline of the ear, shoulder, hip joint (greater trochanter), knee joint (lateral condyle), and ankle joint (lateral malleolus).

The tilt of the pelvis from the Posterior Superior Iliac Spine (PSIS) and Anterior Superior Iliac Spine (ASIS) is the same (optimally at 10 degrees). Looking from the front view (Sagittal Plane), the spine is straight with no lateral shifts, the legs are straight (knee joints in line with the hip joint and ankle and pointing straight ahead), and the feet balanced (neither collapsed nor rolled out). From the back view (Transverse Plane), the pelvis and the shoulders are level.

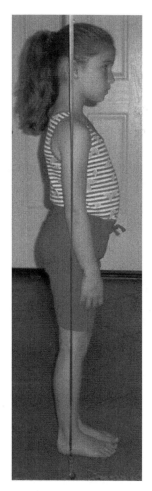

In 2004, we implemented a study at the Explorer Elementary School in San Diego to find out two things. The first was to verify my initial findings of children holding themselves according to the Planes of Motion, and the second was to find out what age-group started to show misalignment leading them away from this ideal blueprint. Our findings were astonishing, which revealed the main reason why we have so much pain in our world today.

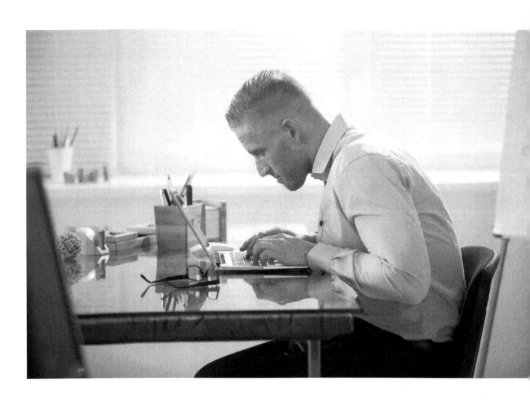

"Sitting, in my opinion, is the number one reason we have chronic pain."

~ Patrick Mummy

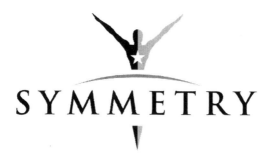

SYMMETRY

CAUSES OF MISALIGNMENT

Now that we have established that gravity exists, and that our bodies rely on this force to stand upright, then movement is the key to keeping ourselves healthy and happy. However, our environment is terrible regarding keeping us healthy and happy because we stop having proper movement at such an early age. Think about it this way. Has technology helped or hindered us? Not so long ago, I was at a restaurant and observed a family of five sitting at a table near me. There were three kids ranging from around 3 to 8, each one intently focused on their anti-social devices (ASDs). I am sure they are on these ASDs at home as well when they should be out playing in the back yard. When I was growing up, we did not have portable devices, PlayStations, or X-Boxes. Atari had just come out, but you had to have plenty of disposable income to afford one. I tell my kids that I remember growing up with a black and white television and we had to get up to change the channel. Today, we live in a different era due to the amount of technology we are privy to have at our fingertips. Most parents today are more than willing to shut their kids up and out. Are we really surprised that our country leads the world in the number of obese children? Children today simply do not move like my friends and I did as children. My mom had to yell at me to get inside after dark.

Then, there is education. What age were you when you started school? On average, we all start school around five years old, and we also begin to sit. Previously I discussed the concept "form follows function". This is true for a well-functioning society where we continue to move 80% of the day our entire lives. However, because we stop moving consistently at such an early age, the intrinsic holding patterns around an extended and balanced body begin to regress, and the older we get, the more chairs we find ourselves in on a regular basis.

What we found in our research at Explorer Elementary, was that nine-year-olds already show significant misalignments. At a time when the body needs movement more than ever to support our natural design, we place kids in a desk, which impedes the natural process of keeping the body upright and extended. Therefore, sitting, in my opinion, is the number one reason we have chronic pain. Our intrinsic muscles are attached in a specific, strategic way to hold our frame in its optimal orthogonal position, otherwise known as the Planes of Motion. When we sit, our frame is in its most flexed position which completely de-emphasizes the intrinsic integrity response. We were designed to be able to sit, but not for long periods of time. And the more time we sit, the less integrity our intrinsic muscles have. In fact, when we sit, we literally shut off two out of three planes of muscles because we are sitting. The Frontal Plane muscles only function when one is standing, as their responsibility is to support the body laterally and medially in a static position, much like the lateral stabilizers of the Golden Gate Bridge. If these cables were taken out of the design of this bridge, the bridge itself would sag down towards the water. In much the same way, if we don't use the lateral/medial Frontal Plane muscles by not standing and moving as we should, then when we do attempt to stand up, our pelvis is thrust forward due to the lack of stability within these muscle groups.

The Transverse Plane muscle group is also shut off because when we are sitting on our pelvis, the insertions of the rotational muscles in the pelvis have no effect on stabilizing through the torso because again, there is no extension while sitting through the pelvis and legs. In her book, *Sitting Kills, Moving Heals*, Joan Vernikos Ph.D., the former director of NASA's Life Science Division, validated the conclusion of comparing sitting to that of being weightless in space. It only takes up to 72-hours of non-loadbearing positioning to start negatively affecting the anti-gravitational muscles (intrinsic), thereby supporting the theory that if you don't use it, you lose it. Think about your life for a moment. You went to school at the age of five, sat the majority of your educational life, only to graduate from college to get a job where you either sit all day long or stand in one position for long periods of time. The fact remains that even if you have a functional job as an adult, you already have had nearly 20 years of incorrect patterning due to not using your body as it was intended. Once you have developed that patterning, unless you are specifically intentional on correcting it, your body adds one layer at a time, one year at a time, and never lets it go. Eventually your body will give up or give out and you are left with a chronic situation that you are not sure how to reverse.

At this point, the adage "form follows function" becomes reversed, because if you are standing out of alignment, then you are going to move out of alignment, which only strengthens these compensation patterns. What needs to be addressed first is the dysfunctional holding pattern of the body so that when you move, you are moving effectively and efficiently around the force of gravity. Therefore, function must follow form, otherwise you will continue to exacerbate the misalignments accrued over your lifetime and nothing will change relative to your symptoms. It would be remarkably like your car being out of alignment and your tires wearing out unevenly. If you do not fix the misalignment, then new tires will wear in the same exact fashion.

The next main cause of misalignment is due to injury. I remember when I was in high school and I fractured my ankle playing basketball. For six weeks, I was on crutches until my ankle healed and then I was back to my normal activities. I was a running back in high school football, getting tackled 20 times per game. I once calculated that I literally crashed on average every five yards nearly 500 times over my high school career. In college, I was always getting injured, the worst pain I ever felt was taking a foul ball off my tibia. When we suffer an injury, we do not think of the consequences that result from not having normal activity during the period your body recovers. Every time we put our bodies in a long-term situation of non-activity, the body must adjust, meaning we compensate. What we do not realize is that in the same way sitting causes decreased intrinsic function, so does using our body in a unilateral way for a long period of time as we recover from an injury.

Six weeks is a long enough time to incorporate imbalance and misalignment in the body due to avoiding the injured site. Think about how many injuries you have sustained over your lifetime, each one adding a layer of compensation and misalignment. When we are working with a client, one thing that often happens is the reintroduction of old symptoms from a specific prior accident or injury. The reason this happens is because when we originally had the injury, we never rehabbed our whole body back to balance; we just worked on the area that was injured. The compensation that initiated from the injury never really leaves the body when the injured site is healed and ultimately, chronic pain is the result of our history of injuries and compensations.

In my case, my injuries were consistent, at least the ones that were non-contact. I always sprained my left ankle, right quad and left hamstring; my right sacroiliac (SI) joint would always go out, and I had chronic Plantar Fasciitis in both feet. Whenever I would get an injury, I would go to the training room already knowing the exact treatment protocol that would be used. What bothered me the most with respect to the recurring injuries I would sustain, was the consistent lack of understanding about what I could do to prevent these injuries from happening again and again. In retrospect, I realize that the symptom was being treated and not the cause. So even though the injury would eventually heal, I was taking the same misaligned body back onto the playing field.

Repetitive stress is the next reason for misalignment. Let us recap our discussion to this current point. It takes you at least one year to stand and move from the time you are born. We then spend the next three years playing, running, jumping, and twisting. Never sitting still for long periods. Then, we get thrusted into pre-K and then kindergarten, and we take most of the movement out of our lives. Then, on to grade school, high school, and college. We sit more and more the higher the educational demand. Why? To graduate and get a job so we can sit some more or get a job that has us in dysfunctional positions all day. But we are not just sitting or standing. We add a computer in front of us with a mouse, or we stand and bend over patients all day in awkward positions.

Either way, we not only have the previous years of compensations to contend with, but now we enter a profession that adds to the dysfunction. We literally become what we do. Akin to the clichéd expression "we are what we eat". Daily habits imposed on the body start to imprint negative structural patterns. However, it does not stop at this point. For those of us who still want to be active, we take our misaligned bodies into our activities and do not realize that we are simply adding to the dysfunction. As I mentioned in the first chapter, when I was a senior in college prior to my last season of baseball, I lived in the weight room. I went from bench-pressing 200 pounds to 300 pounds in three months. What I did not understand is that my misaligned body was still misaligned while I was lifting, and therefore all I was doing was making my dysfunctions stronger. I know for a fact that this was the leading contributor to my increased injuries that year.

Furthermore, whenever I stretched, I always felt worse. Why? Because I was stretching out the tight muscles. Up until now, logic dictates that stretching out tight muscles would be a natural focal point to getting out of pain, right? Wrong! Tight muscles, as we will learn shortly, are there to provide some type of stability to an imbalanced frame. We will be talking much more about compensation and how that intertwines with pain and performance, but for now, understand that your repetitive stress on an imbalanced frame is causing more and more imbalance. What this simply means is that your daily, monthly, and yearly habits continually add to your imbalanced frame unless you prepare your body for each daily routine that you start for yourself. So, stretching, for the sake of stretching, and without the combination of some type of strengthening, can result in more pain or create injury.

Sports dominance is another cause of misalignment. In the 25 years of experiencing postural dysfunctions, we have come across thousands of athletes. There is no better explanation of "you are what you do" than to look at sports and how it creates bad habits. In 2003, I was at the Las Vegas airport with my wife and we passed by a college team waiting to board their plane. They were all wearing their team gear, but it was not clear exactly what type of team they were. I turned to my wife and explained to her that they were the swim team, and to my surprise she made a bet that I was wrong! So, she went up to one of the members and asked, and came back with a grimace on her face, because I was right!

In 2004, I was flown up to the University of Washington (UW) to work with Steve Emtman who was the strength and conditioning coach for UW at the time. For you football fans, Steve was drafted number one overall by the Indianapolis Colts in 1992 as a Defensive End. Steve had been my very first student with my Symmetry Core certification program in 2001 and when he was given the job at UW, he and I immediately talked about getting his athletes aligned. What was remarkably interesting was when I worked with the different teams, it was very apparent how their patterns were developed due to the different type of sport in which they were involved. In Track and field, sprinters were very Frontal Plane deviated and hurdlers were very Transverse Plane deviated. Swimmers were very Frontal Plane deviated, which is why I could tell at the Las Vegas airport that the team we saw was indeed the swim team. You see, when we look at swimmers, the first thing we must understand is that we weigh 10% of our body weight when in the pool. Spending hours in the water automatically shuts off the intrinsic muscular system as it pertains to dealing with gravity. There is no vertical loadbearing taking place while swimming, therefore the strength that occurs is almost strictly dynamic as one moves through the water. Due to this lack of vertical loadbearing, the Frontal Plane muscle groups are extremely limited in their recruitment as they mainly function in standing postures. When I observed the swim team at the airport, their sport posture was very obvious to me because when looking at their profiles, their hips and head were very forward, trapezium very enlarged and engaged, and latissimus dorsi very developed as well.

Az Hakim was part of the "Greatest Show on Turf" when he played with the St. Louis Rams during their Super Bowl season in 1999-2000. As mentioned in the foreword, I met him in 2004 when I was introduced to him by the former New York Giant and coach, Harland Svare, with whom we worked with intimately. At this point in his career, Az was picked up by the New Orleans Saints and during pre-season he suffered multiple pulls of his hamstring. One day Az called me and told me that the trainers with the Saints were not addressing his real issues, because all they were doing was treating his hamstring. One of the issues most athletes develop is related to their strength training. If 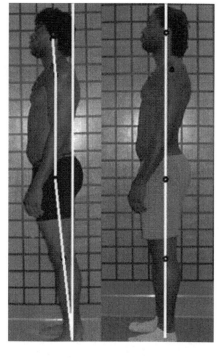 you look at the first picture of Az, you will see how forward he is. When most athletes take time to strength train, they work mainly in the Sagittal Plane, meaning that almost every movement in the weight room is linear, consisting of flexion and extension. From the bench press to the squat, athletes are disproportionately training by working primarily in one plane, which decreases structural stability and alignment in the other two planes.

What ends up happening is that the weaker the Frontal plane becomes, the harder it is for the body to hold itself upright and aligned in the Frontal Plane (laterally). As the body becomes weaker in the Frontal Plane and stronger in the Sagittal Plane, the more forward the hips move, thus prompting a response from the hamstrings in order to keep the body from falling over. Hence the true issue is weakness in the frontal plane which provokes a compensatory tightness in the hamstring, which is a deviation in the Sagittal Plane. The hamstrings are recruited by the brain to literally keep the body from falling over, so when an athlete proceeds with treatment only around pain or tightness, such as the hamstring in Az's case, nothing will release long term if the initial cause is not addressed.

Az flew me out to the Saint's facility after pulling his hamstring for the third time, and after one postural alignment treatment, he was out running the next day, and in full gear four days later. He never had a hamstring pull again.

Genetics is the last reason for misalignment. Although this diagnosis, in my opinion, is handed out too frequently, there are cases that directly or indirectly lead to the body not being aligned. However, you must determine whether genetics truly causes misalignment or not. In some scoliotic cases, this will absolutely lead to misalignment. But there are two types of scoliosis, so one must rule out which one is genetic, and which one is a product of your environment, known as functional scoliosis.

Many times, I get clients in that say they have been diagnosed with a leg-length discrepancy. I am here to tell you that this is just not as prevalent as you might think. The only true way you can determine if one has a leg-length discrepancy is through x-rays, and then measuring the length of each individual leg bones. However, even with that accomplished, you are still not considering joint compression and compensation in all planes that may affect the overall loadbearing instability. One cannot lay a patient on a table, wiggle the legs a few times, and show you a picture of one foot further than the other to properly determine whether one leg is longer than the other.

The picture you see here is of a 14-year-old client named Hannah, who was diagnosed with scoliosis. Her doctor wanted to fuse her entire spine, but her parents wisely took her to another doctor who recommended Symmetry. What you see is the change we made on the first session! Yes, Hannah has structural scoliosis, but the level of functional scoliosis as a result, was very much changeable. Regardless of what you have been told, your body can change.

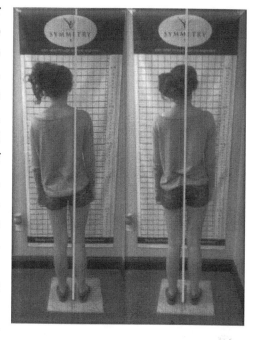

In any case, do not let a diagnosis of genetics set you in a space of blind acceptance as it pertains to the explanation of your chronic pain. Even if you can verify that there is a genetic component to your misalignment, you still have all the prior four reasons that add to this dysfunctional pattern, which still need to be addressed and corrected. Using me as an example, I believe that genetics played a large part of causing my problems. Just look at this picture of me when I was five years old; knees valgus (knock-kneed) and externally rotated, to mention a couple of disparities.

There is no doubt that the body I was given was genetically manipulated. However, I blame it on being the youngest of six kids and getting the remains of the gene pool from my dad. By the way, my dad's name is Gene! I always knew growing up that I was not put together all that well, and that it somehow had to relate to the pains from which I suffered. No one else ever related my faulty structure to my chronic issues, but I knew it was. It really did not matter once I found the solution.

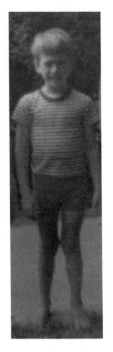

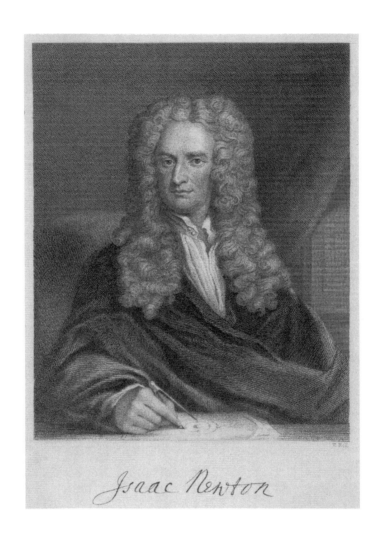

Isaac Newton

"*For every action there is an equal and opposite reaction.*"

~ Isaac Newton

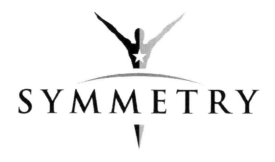

SYMMETRY

THE PHYSICS OF PAIN
(NEWTON'S THIRD LAW)

Symmetry can be defined simply as dealing with gravity and the laws of the universe. Whenever we get a client in front of us, we ask them if anyone has ever explained their pain as it relates to gravity. The answer inevitably is No! This is because we tend to move pain to the forefront of the perceived problem, and therefore, most of the conversation is focused on the pain itself. For example, many of our clients are extremely excited to show us their X-rays or MRI reports. They assume we will also want to talk about these reports because that is what they are used to talking about when dealing with their pain. To us, the pain is simply the by-product of systemic breakdown due to years of dysfunction and not a complete reason in and of itself. Newton's third law states that "For every action there is an equal and opposite reaction". This law is the basis from which Symmetry was created and it remains the most important aspect of Symmetry because we can always depend on gravity.

Gravity is defined as the force of attraction by which terrestrial bodies tend to fall toward the center of the earth. In physics terms, this means that gravity is a constant. Just as an architect designs a building, or an engineer a car, the number one issue he or she focuses on is gravity and the forces that apply to the structures surrounding it, whether static or dynamic. Newton's Laws all pertain to this one phenomenon, but his third law specifically addresses postural deviations because we are focusing on static holding patterns, and thereby we focus on intrinsic muscles. This constant that we count on is twofold because: gravity falls perpendicular to the surface of earth; and, any structure must react directly in opposition to that force in order to hold itself upright and move effectively and efficiently.

When we do not apply the reaction to the force of gravity in a constant and equal way, then any structure will be forced to adjust. This is the definition of compensation. Compensation, therefore, is the intent to improve any defect by the excessive development or action of another structure or organ of the same structure (Wikipedia, 2018). Given the force of gravity, if the foundation of a building is not level or strong enough, then it can be assumed that the walls will be under stress due to this imbalance. When we look at any structure, there is a fundamental understanding of balance that we instinctively take for granted. For example, you assume that your car is aligned properly. You also assume that the building you are in now was constructed correctly and that the walls will not fall on you. We also assume and know instinctively that if these structures are not aligned, then there will be a compensation that will occur, such as a tire that wears unevenly when the alignment is off.

If we were to initially assume that the issue is not with the alignment and solely with the tire, at some point we would question why each new replaced tire is wearing in the exact same way as its predecessor. When we are discussing compensation with regards to our frame, we take the approach in most cases that the pain is not associated with the alignment of the body, or in this case, the misalignment. However, we must understand the nature of compensation and why it occurs in the first place and then relate it to the pain that we feel. Here are two main reasons the body compensates:

- <u>Reason #1</u>. The main reason that the body will compensate is because our sympathetic nervous system is such that pain will be avoided at all costs if the brain detects a weakness or imbalance in our system. Its general action is to mobilize the body's nervous system fight or flight response, which is a physiological reaction that occurs in response to a perceived harmful event or attack, or threat to survival. The body constantly aims to maintain homeostasis, which is derived from the Greek Homeo or constant, and stasis or stable, meaning to remain stable or remaining the same. The human body manages a multitude of extraordinarily complex interactions to maintain balance or return systems to functioning within a normal range. These interactions within the body facilitate compensatory changes supportive of physical and psychological functioning. This process is essential to the survival of the person and to our species.

- <u>Reason #2</u>. The second reason our bodies compensate is due to the righting reflex. "The righting reflex, also known as the labyrinthine righting reflex, is a reflex that corrects the orientation of the body when it is taken out of its normal upright position. It is initiated by the vestibular system (sensory system that is responsible for providing our brain with information about motion, head position, and spatial orientation), which detects that the body is not erect and causes the head to move back into position as the rest of the body follows. The perception of head movement involves the body sensing linear acceleration or the force of gravity through the otoliths, a structure in the saccule of the inner ear and angular acceleration through the semicircular canals. The reflex uses a combination of visual system inputs, vestibular inputs, and somatosensory inputs to make postural adjustments when the body becomes displaced from its normal vertical position.

These inputs are used to create what is called an efference copy. This means that the brain makes comparisons in the cerebellum between expected posture and perceived posture and corrects for the difference." (Wikipedia, 2018)

The righting reflex is one of the biggest examples of compensation and gravity because your eyes must always be level with the horizon to maintain balance and equilibrium. What we have not considered, however, is the fact that once your body becomes structurally misaligned, we spend a lifetime utilizing this reflex to literally keep our heads on straight. The question is not whether the head must be balanced, but what triggers the righting reflex in the first place. This, again, is where Newton's third law comes into effect because the righting reflex is nothing more than Newton's third law in action, because for every compensation there is an equal and opposite physical compensation.

Check out this picture and ask yourself what is the first thing that pops out at you. At first glance you probably will notice how uneven this person's shoulders are as designated by the stripes on her shirt. However, if you look more closely, you will see that her pelvis is also uneven. This is where we must break the body down into its basic parts and explain it in terms of physics. What we must assess is what came first, the chicken or the egg? Did the elevated shoulder come first, or the elevated hip?

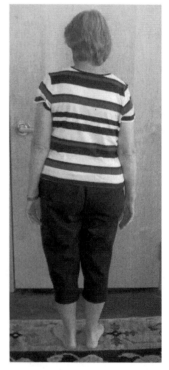

When a client comes into our office, we do not look at them in terms of pain as we have already discussed, but rather as a delicate system of levers and pulleys. Leverage is defined as the mechanical advantage or power gained by using a lever. A lever is defined as a rigid bar resting on a pivot, used to help move a heavy or rigidly fixed load with one end when pressure is applied to the other (i.e. bones). A pulley is defined as a device for overcoming resistance at one point by applying force at some other point (i.e. muscles). Why is this necessary to understand? First, the body works best when it is as extended and balanced as possible in three-dimensional space. We again define this as the Planes of Motion. If the body is in its correct orthogonal position, then all the bones (levers), and all the muscles (pulleys), will be in what we call harmonic tension, which simply means that in the static standing position, all the muscles, both intrinsic and dynamic, are at their proper length, and therefore leveraged to hold and move the body in its most efficient way possible. Plato, in his Theory of Forms, states that "Beauty of form is that which moves with the least amount of energy".

Taking into consideration levers/bones and pulleys/muscles when we are assessing the body, we must break the body down further into two simple parts. The first is the foundation or Locomotor Unit, comprised of the pelvis and legs. The second is the Passenger Unit, comprised of the upper torso. It is important to label the body using these two physics terms because we must begin to understand where leverage is originated in the body and how it relates to pain and gravity. The pelvis, in our research, is the most important part of the body because this is where the line of gravity should bisect the body. It is further defined by the Center of Mass (COM), which is the unique point where the weighted relative position of the distributed mass sums to zero, or true balance. So, how does Symmetry define COM? It is defined simply by the Planes of Motion.

If you take the Transverse, Frontal and Sagittal planes and assess where they intersect, this represents the COM. Theoretically, if you are completely aligned along all three planes, then the COM should be located at the second or third sacral joint, or just superior of the acetabulum (hip joint). In most studies of the COM of the human body, the results are located much higher than this, usually in the lumbar or in some studies, the lower thoracic region. The reason for this is because we spend the majority of our lives sitting, and what we had mentioned previously is that when we sit, we completely disengage the frontal plane muscle group because there is no response for stability of these muscles while sitting. Then, when we do stand, due to the inactivity and weakness of these muscles, the pelvis is thrust forward due to lack of lateral stabilization, thus the COM is forced upwards initiating a completely different weighted relative position of the distributed mass. The upper body, or the Passenger Unit, is then forced to rebalance back in order to sustain the righting reflex, which can be further defined as not only rebalancing the head, but rebalancing the head back over the pelvis, as this is the true aspect of how equilibrium works.

In other words, your brain not only has to have the head level through the use of sight, but also cannot ultimately stabilize itself without proprioceptively balancing itself over the pelvis, as the brain instinctively knows that in order to move anywhere, this relationship must be intact. So, as the pelvis is thrust forward in the above analogy, and the torso is rebalanced back, the head must then reposition back over the pelvis, which is the basic posture you see with people who sit for a career. The spine gets caught in the middle of this balancing act. This is not what the spine was intended to do. The purpose of the spine is NOT to support the entire body. This is the main reason most people in the world suffer from lower back pain.

Now, taking into consideration that the Locomotor Unit is responsible for carrying the Passenger Unit, and that the COM is very critical, then there is a reason almost all children up to the age of nine have a 10-degree pelvic tilt. From a leverage standpoint, the 10-degree pelvic tilt creates an optimal holding position for all joints three-dimensionally, supporting the harmonic tension that I previously explained and allowing for the spine to be positioned optimally as well. If you look at the lateral view of the spine, it is composed in such a way as to perform two main functions: provide protection for the nervous system; and, provide support for the Passenger Unit. If the tilt of the pelvis is more than 10-degrees, then the lower spine and above becomes too extended. If the tilt of the pelvis is less than 10-degrees, then the lower spine and above becomes too flexed. Either way it leads to compression, which is causally related to almost ALL diagnoses given regarding back pain. In fact, if you suffer from pain in any joint, you can be assured that you are compressed or compromised in that joint or joints.

Let us check back in with our subject again and go back to the question of the chicken or the egg. Symmetry provides a way to determine when the COM is compromised because we are not using our foundation the way it was intended. Therefore, what begins to break down first is the integrity and balance of the Locomotor Unit. This is due to our environmental miscues and lack of consistent movement from an early age that is required to keep the homeostasis between the Locomotor Unit and the Passenger Unit. Again, the adage "form follows function" was true in our early years, but because we lose function at an early age, form also begins to lose function as well. If we simply take a subject and try to start moving it more, the form still stays dysfunctional and therefore tends to exacerbate the structural compensations with movement.

> *The purpose of the spine is NOT to support the entire body. This is the main reason most people in the world suffer from lower back pain.*

Look at the woman in the striped shirt. Using Symmetry, we determined that her compensations began mainly with the imbalance of the pelvis or Locomotor Unit in the Transverse Plane, which causes the reaction of the righting reflex. This is the case for most clients. In her case, the elevation of the left hip caused an offset of the lumbar

49

spine towards the elevated hip, which caused the reaction of her left shoulder to elevate to reposition her head. When assessing one's posture, ultimately, we must determine which plane we must address first to correct years of accrued dysfunction. This is the basis for which we were awarded a patent, allowing us to create a personalized and evolving sequence of the isometric stretches and strengthening positions that are derived from 20 specific measurements taken at each visit. The before and after pictures you see here are from the first session. Her issues were two bulged discs in her neck, with radiating pain down her arm, and her doctor wanted to perform surgery. However, since Symmetry does not focus solely on pain, we went after the cause. You can see that in the after picture, her shoulders are much more level, even though we did not directly treat the upper body. She came in with a level of eight on the pain scale and left with a level of two and never had the surgery her doctor recommended. At first she couldn't understand why we didn't treat her neck like everyone had done previously, but when she was through with her routine, she understood why it worked and that now she had access to a long-term solution with the tools and support we provided to her.

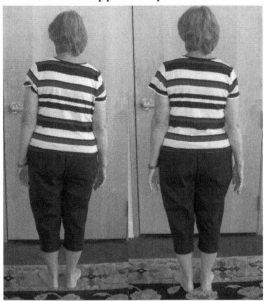

In another case, the pictures you see next, are of a client (Jim) who came in four months after a hip-replacement. He was still in pain and walking with a limp, but the pain was now in his lower back and not his hip. I showed him this Frontal Plane view and asked him what was wrong with this picture. In his beautiful British accent, he said, "I never realized my head was that bloody forward!" To this day, I am still amazed by the surprised reactions clients have to their photos, given that other treatments never highlighted their misalignments.

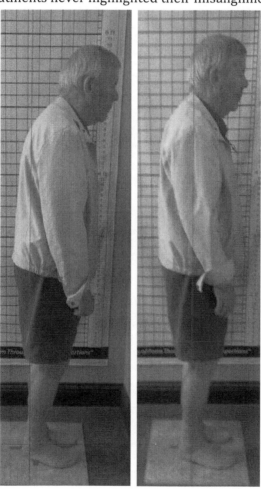

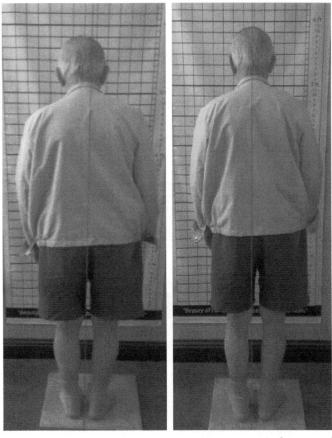

Whenever I give a seminar to practitioners, I always ask who in the room takes pictures of their clients, whether for the first session or at each session. I am lucky if I see two hands raised. The next question I ask is "Why don't you?". Mostly I get the answer, "Because we were never taught to!". I already know what the answer is going to be, because client participation is not the priority in higher education. Most of what practitioners learn is how to treat a patient or client, rather than how to teach them to treat themselves. It is the old proverb about fishing; you can give a person a fish and momentarily satiate their hunger, or you can teach that person to fish, which is the more sustainable solution. Generally, there is no real incentive to show people what they look like after treatment, because the common emphasis is to focus on how they feel after a treatment. Our philosophy at Symmetry is to not only show clients their postural progress from session to session, but more importantly, to measure their progress from session to session. If you have never looked at yourself in the mirror, you might want to take a closer look. You could even have someone take pictures of you and look to see what is true about your own posture. Later, we will give you steps to check your own posture and see how you compare to three-dimensional alignment!

Now, let us talk more about our British client. This is a 75-year-old man who had a complete left hip replacement. You saw his profile and how forward his load-bearing joints were, from head to knee. Again, in physics terminology, we are attuning to the center of mass concept. I had mentioned that when properly aligned, the COM should be around S2-3 or slightly lower. When our static posture starts to deviate away from its planar stability points, then this directly affects the COM. Look at his before back picture. Just using your own subjective eye, which leg do you think he is leaning more onto? Which hip do you think was replaced? If you answered, the left hip, then you would be correct!

When you add his profile picture along with this posterior view, you will determine that the way the body must hold itself up due to his compensation pattern is mainly through his left side and lower than normal COM, in other words, his left hip. You see, when we compensate over a lifetime, our body tends to wear out at the point of the COM adjustment, or where the body has reacted the most to these compensations to help balance out the body. As I mentioned previously, most people suffer from lower back issues because the back is doing way more work than it was designed to perform. In this case, Jim compensated in a way that forced him to use his left hip more than it was intended. However, the left hip is the victim of his compensation pattern, not the cause. Once Jim got his left hip replaced, you can see in these pictures that the same misaligned frame still existed. Therefore, the same compensation patterns were still occurring, and he still landed more heavily on his left hip, which is why he still had pain, but now in his back!

My biggest argument with surgery is not related to the surgery itself, but the lack of patient preparation prior to surgery. I call it prehab. You see, many surgeons are trained in surgery, not physics. Therefore, when they show you the MRI or X-rays, and tell you that the reason you have pain is clearly diagnosed, they fail to tell you that your entire body has completely compensated for the reasons stated in the chapter, Causes of Misalignment. It is this compensation which has led to your specific problem, because of the reaction your body had to your misalignments.

Perhaps you have the procedure done, and a day or week later you feel better because the pressure on the nerve was relieved, but your tires are still going to wear out because your frame is still off. When we get clients in to see us who are on track for surgery, our first intent is to prevent the surgery, and we have succeeded many times. However, even if the surgery cannot be avoided, the body's compensations need to be fixed prior to the surgery so that the recovery is easier and more importantly, to avoid future surgeries! Again, we call this prehab. Check out Jim's first-session pictures, after just 20-minutes of the AlignSmart™ exercises.

The real interesting thing about this first routine is that I kept Jim on the floor in a supine position throughout the entire sequence. One of the factors we use to determine the proper sequencing of a corrective exercise routine is called ramping. It is equivalent to what I previously discussed about the development process from birth to standing, and how our individual process mimics this patterning. Sometimes I get clients who are just too compensated and cannot get off the floor due to the complexity of their dysfunctions. I do not mean that they literally cannot get off the floor. In Jim's case, he clearly walked into our clinic on his first visit and walked out of our clinic when he was through with his visit. What I mean is if I had taken him off the floor during his initial corrective sequence, the entire connection would have been lost because his patterning was too engrained. Remember the levers and pulleys? If you try and rebuild the structure too fast, it will always default to its defensive point, or the state that feels the safest, even if that state is dysfunctional. Jim left much more aligned even though I did not take him off the floor during his treatment routine.

In the following chapters I am going to lay out a more comprehensive technical explanation of physics, gravity, compensation, and its effects on our structure, which I have only hinted at in previous chapters. These chapters set the stage for a more in-depth explanation of how Symmetry's AlignSmart™ system works and why I was awarded a patent for this technology.

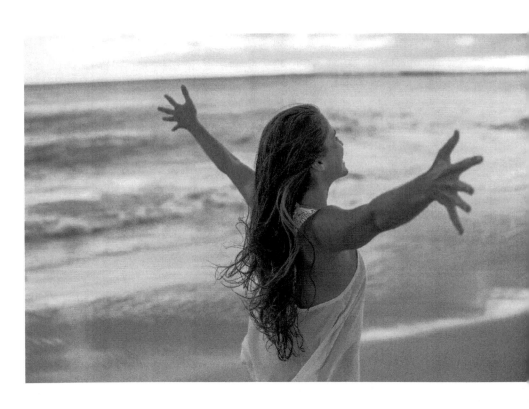

"Better than 90% of the brain's output is directed toward maintaining your body in its gravitational field. Therefore, the less one spends on one's posture, the more energy is available for healing, digestion, and thinking."

~ Roger Sperry
Neuropsychologist, Nobel Prize Winner

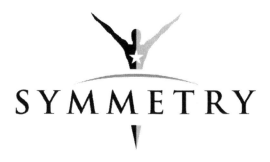

SYMMETRY

BENEFITS OF STRUCTURAL ALIGNMENT

Structural alignment is important because we live on Planet Earth, which is subject to the constant downward force of gravity, as we have discussed. To balance erect on two limbs on Earth's surface we must counter the downward forces and do so in the most efficient manner possible. The primary focus of our existence should not be battling gravity. Yet without realizing it, this is what most of us are spending our energy doing. Symmetry's Postural Alignment Technology™ program is designed to reinstate our structural integrity, thereby freeing up our energy for other types of activities and functions that help develop our lives so we can progress as a species on this planet.

Importance of Structural Alignment

The erect posture is a result of a very dynamic process of checks and balances. It is what is achieved when the various systems of the body, including the skeletal, muscular, and nervous systems, are in balance with each other and the external environment. However, this is not a static state. Therefore, our ability to stand erect is a continual process of adaptation to both internal and external stimuli.

Structural alignment is defined as skeletal correctness in the human body. It is essentially what is achieved when the skeletal frame is positioned perpendicular to the earth's surface and the force of gravity. This right-angle (90-degree) relationship between our body and the environment forms the criterion for both anatomical and physiological correctness, as well as psychological and emotional well-being. When this right-angle fundamental is achieved, the skeletal system operates at its highest level, achieving the most amount of work with the least amount of effort. As we have established, anatomical correctness is when the three planes of the body divide the body equally to form right angles at all eight load bearing joints. This will position the body perpendicular to the Earth's surface, which will enable the skeleton to carry most of the body's weight with minimal muscular tension.

Physiological correctness is when the organ systems of the body operate effectively and efficiently. In other words, the organs are spaced sufficiently apart to receive adequate nutrition (i.e. water, oxygen, minerals, and vitamins) from the circulatory system, and expand and contract maximally. This can only be achieved if the body is in a state of anatomical correctness. For example, the inter-relatedness of physiological and anatomical correctness can be readily observed by the effect of posture on the heart.

One of the axial skeleton's purposes is to house and protect our organ system. Every organ is packed into this bony casing like a jigsaw puzzle, with every piece fitting perfectly against the next. There is no room for anything else. Organ walls consist of a labyrinth of veins and arteries that carry nourishment to, and waste away from their cells. Any skeletal misalignment leads to compensation. Compensation, in this context, means that the space that these organs fit into is changing. Should the change be one of decreased space (as in the prevalent rounded shoulder posture/kyphosis) the result will be organ crowding. Organ crowding inhibits the ability of the lungs to expand fully and take in enough oxygen. It cannot, therefore, provide adequate oxygen to the rest of the organ systems, which include the heart. If the heart is undernourished, it will be weak and unable to pump enough blood to the brain and the body. Without adequate oxygen and nutrients carried in the blood, the various organ systems will soon become undernourished and weak, and their tissue will begin to atrophy and die. Cardiovascular Disease (CVD) results from a combination of factors, but all are aspects of organ crowding and inability of body organs to perform their intended job function.

In summary, when the bones are not perpendicular to the Earth's surface and the line of gravity, an optimal internal environment, where the organ systems of the body can operate 100% effectively and efficiently, cannot be maintained. Nor can the skeleton carry most of the body's weight with minimal muscular tension. What this means is that our body will hold excess tension in and around its load bearing joints, leaving the organ systems too weak and undernourished. These compromised physical states severely inhibit our ability to live our lives completely; the fundamental inhibiting factor being fatigue and subsequent weakness.

Our corporeal (relating to a physical material body) energy system is a closed system. What this means is that we have a limited amount of internally derived energy, and only so much more that can be created from external sources such as food. In the human body, all things are not considered equal. Therefore, functions of more importance for survival, such as our heart pumping, will be given higher priority and afforded more energy if required. For example, if Mr. Joe is having a heart attack, all his available energy will be directed towards coping with the sudden change in status quo and in the reestablishment of homeostasis. It doesn't matter how long ago he ate or what deadlines at work he was thinking about; he will not feel hungry nor will he continue to think about work. His body has a new priority, which is to get enough blood pumped out of his heart to his brain. The same would be true if Mr. Joe's posture resembled that of the letter C, a clear representation of Kyphotic Posture. This posture demonstrates an anterior/posterior imbalance, which can also be called Frontal Plane deviation; it results in the inability of the body to maintain its right angle fundamental and remain perpendicular to the Earth's surface. This is the most efficient position for the human body.

What this means is that Mr. Joe should be able to walk, sit, and think with minimal muscular effort. However, this is not the situation. A lot of Mr. Joe's energy will go to his muscular and skeletal systems as both attempts to reestablish anterior/posterior homeostasis. Over time, if Mr. Joe does not do anything to improve his situation and his posture remains the same, then reestablishing energy requirement will increase. Not only will it become harder to stand and move, but in addition his various other systems will become less and less efficient and eventually cease operating due to atrophy and a lack of adequate nutrition. Disorders of the digestive system and colon can be pervasive in clients with kyphosis due to organ crowding and the fact that the body perceives activities such as digestion to be less important, from a basic survival perspective, than standing erect, moving, and breathing.

Roger Sperry won the Nobel Prize for physiology of medicine for his discoveries concerning the functional specialization of the cerebral hemispheres. The summary of his work is described in this quote, "Better than 90% of the brain's output is directed toward maintaining your body in its gravitational field. Therefore, the less one spends on one's posture, the more energy is available for healing, digestion and thinking."

Example: A Sprained Ankle

Previously I mentioned that I broke my ankle in high school and sprained my ankle numerous times in college playing baseball. Every time this happened to me, the affected ankle joint was unable to be utilized as a load bearing structure. Therefore, it could no longer provide for absorption and dispersion of ground reaction forces, nor could it act as the fulcrum for the foot lever, which is the mechanism by which the body propels itself forward or walk, as it is more commonly known. This means that the affected ankle has led to the entire system being unable to perform its most fundamental and unique function, that of bipedal ambulation. This lack of functioning, both muscularly and skeletally, will affect all contingent systems such as the circulatory, endocrine, and lymph systems that rely on the equal use and distribution of gravity to perform their functions. What this demonstrates is that skeletal correctness affects us on a physical level. However, skeletal correctness can also affect us emotionally and psychologically. The restoration of physical balance and function within a person provides stability in the physical realm, thereby facilitating choices of how they respond to physical, mental, emotional, and energetic challenges (Gluckman, 1998).

Today, a 60-hour workweek is commonplace, as is driving a car, traveling, going to the movies, and working out. Stop and think for a minute how you would feel if you could not sit for more than 20-minutes without experiencing excruciating pain. How would this impact your life and how would you feel about yourself and your life? We see many clients who have not been to the movies, or traveled, or had sex in years. These clients report feeling out of control, frustrated, and depressed. In addition, their bodies hold these feelings and manifest them physically. The postural evaluations I perform while applying Symmetry allow me to observe the emotional stance of a person. It is an opportunity to visually and auditorily assess the messages coming from a client.

The example of an ankle sprain is only a minor disruption of homeostasis. Therefore, it should if logic prevails, only lead to minor compensations within the system. However, if you have ever sprained your ankle you know there is nothing minor about it. Yet, in the scheme of possible compensation and dysfunction, a sprained ankle is still considered minor. One can, therefore, imagine the level of compensation the body must undergo, and subsequent fatigue it will suffer, in order to cope with disorders such as scoliosis, kyphosis, or spina bifida, which are disorders of the axial skeleton and, therefore, affect the system at its core structural level.

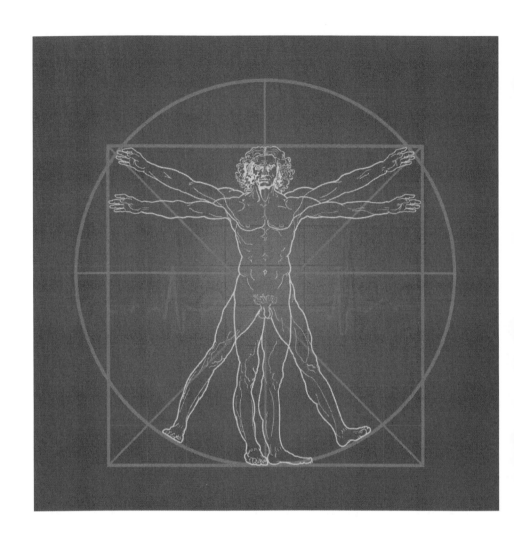

"Regardless of theory and opinion, the human body is an amazing design."

~ *Patrick Mummy*

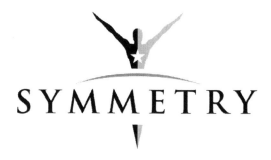

SYMMETRY

THE PHYSICS OF RIGHT ANGLES

The goal of Postural Alignment Technology™ is to reestablish the body's balance and function in reference to the force of gravity, and to return it to its ability for movement in all planes and ranges of motion. This will return the body to being bilateral with the left side being a mirror image of the right side. From a skeletal structure perspective, this will occur when every load bearing joint, namely the ankles, knees, hips, and shoulders, lies in parallel horizontal relation to each other and to the ground, in healthy relation to the plumb line of gravity. These joints should all face forward, and therefore produce three dimensional right angles. These right angles will then be able to distribute forces equally to the appropriate structures. When such bilateralism is achieved, and movement is restored, large forces, upwards of 100 times one's body weight, can be quite easily managed by the body without excessive strain, attrition, or pain.

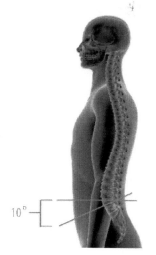

Previously I mentioned that the optimal pelvic tilt is 10 degrees, which is what we found in measuring hundreds of children up to the age of 9 years old. The reason this makes sense is that when you analyze the spine in its purest form, in young children, the angle of the PSIS to ASIS has a 90-degree angle in relation to the fourth lumbar vertebra through to the second sacral joint. This creates the most effective position for the lower lumbar vertebrae to support the entire spine on top of the pelvis, in terms of both shock absorption and nerve protection. Anything less than 10 degrees in the pelvic tilt will cause too much flexion in the lower lumbar spine, which will echo through the thoracic and cervical spine as well. Anything more than a 10 degree tilt of the pelvis will cause too much extension in the lumbar spine, and the effects of this will also carry through to the thoracic and cervical spine. Again, as we previously discussed, if the pelvic tilt is less or more than 10 degrees, the spine will compress on itself which ultimately leads to pain regardless of the diagnosis you are given. This angle produces the optimum leverage for the Passenger Unit to sit on top of the Locomotor Unit to produce the Harmonic Tension we previously discussed.

It is especially important to acknowledge that the real indication of true bilateralism is not so much skeletal perfection, but the ability for the body to be supported as efficiently as possible around the force of gravity. Some experts argue that there is no such thing as true symmetry in the human body, but I argue that within our first five years of life, we are as close to symmetrical as possible and thereafter our negative environmental cues cause a distortion in the developmental process, related back to when we discussed causes of misalignment.

Given that Postural Alignment Technology™ works to reeducate the neurological system, we must focus on neurological output to test for bilateralism. What this means is that if there is equal (bilateral) muscular function, for example, the flexor muscles of both forearms are functioning neurologically the same, then we can say that we have neutralized and balanced the body. Up until now, we have been talking about segmental alignment of the joints from a three-dimensional perspective.

Now, let us put these concepts into the body as a living, breathing, moving human being. During movement, the body functionally divides itself into the Passenger and Locomotor units. While there is motion and muscle action occurring in each function, the relative intensity is markedly different in the two units. Basically, the Passenger Unit is responsible only for its own postural integrity, and when structurally aligned on top of the Locomotor Unit, it has minimal demand. In fact, it should be a relative passive entity that is carried by the Locomotor Unit.

Locomotor Unit

The two lower limbs (legs) and pelvis are the anatomical segments that form the locomotor system. Fifty-seven muscles acting in a selective fashion control timeliness and magnitude of motion in each limb. The bony segments serve as levers. The pelvis has a dual role as the mobile link between the two lower limbs, and the bottom segment of the Passenger Unit that rides on the hips. As the Locomotor Unit carries the body to its desired location, each weight-bearing limb accomplishes five distinct functions:

1. A propulsive force is generated,
2. Upright stability is maintained,
3. The shock of floor impact at the onset of each stride is minimized,
4. Energy is conserved by these functions being performed in a manner that reduces the amount of muscular effort required; and,
5. This Locomotor Unit moves us forward along the surface of the earth, a process known as ambulation.

Passenger Unit

The head, neck, trunk, and arms comprise the Passenger Unit. Muscle action within the neck and trunk serve only to maintain neutral vertebral alignment. Arm swing is both active and passive, but the action does not appear essential to the normal gate pattern (Perry, 1992). Together these four structures make up 70% of a person's body weight. Here is where I disagree with common research. Most experts believe that within this composite mass lies the body's COM located just anterior to the tenth thoracic vertebra. As I have hinted about already, the problem I see with this is that the COM should be located at the sacral level, if not as low as the superior border of the acetabulum because the COM is typically associated with the greatest amount of work being done in a structure. This common conclusion of a higher COM is due to the fact that almost everyone who is analyzed, structurally falls forward at the pelvic level in the Frontal Plane, thus, the work would naturally displace itself higher above the pelvis in order to maintain stability in the body.

This is the reason why most people suffer from lower back pain because the Passenger Unit was not designed to take on the responsibility of holding up the entire body around gravity. As I explained, when we sit for long periods each day and throughout our lives, the lateral and medial stabilizers begin to shorten and become weak and therefore cannot hold the body aligned in the Frontal Plane. So, the natural tendency is for the workload to be transferred higher in the body and into the Passenger Unit in order to maintain some type of balance and homeostasis. However, conventional thought places the COM at a higher level, thereby presenting a long lever above the level of the hip joints. As a result, balance of the Passenger Unit would be even more dependent on the alignment of the lower limbs to move the base of support under the Passenger Unit's momentary center of gravity.

In my opinion, this Passenger Unit is not supposed to be as active during ambulation as traditionally believed. It is supposed to be a more passive unit balancing on top of the Locomotor Unit, which further supports my theory that the COM should be located more in the Locomotor Unit than in the Passenger Unit; one could say it is merely along for the ride. With only one spinal column, this vertical axis provides an efficient counterbalance with the natural gait pattern of two legs flexing and extending at the hip joints.

However, what happens when the Locomotor Unit is either too weak or imbalanced to work, or when it is prevented from doing its work? What we see is that as the strength and amount of work the Locomotor Unit can do diminishes, the role and responsibilities of the Passenger Unit increase in direct relation. If this role reversal exists and persists over an extended period, the size and/or strength of the Passenger Unit will increase to the extent that it will become more imbalanced and thus heavier than normal from its base, the Locomotor Unit, thus destabilizing the unit as a whole. The Passenger Unit under normal circumstances is 70% heavier than the Locomotor Unit, but when asked to do more work due to misalignment or weakness of the Locomotor Unit, the result is that gravity and ground reaction forces no longer meet in the center of the skeletal structure. This leaves both units vulnerable to external forces.

The Passenger Unit now has no counteracting upward force to gravity's downward pulling force. What this means is that the Passenger Unit begins to topple over and move in the direction of gravity's pull, toward the ground. If left to continue, this situation will severely impact both the musculoskeletal and organ systems of the body. The result will be skeletal contortion, excessive strain and attrition on the bones, muscles and all soft tissue structures, generalized or chronic pain and discomfort, vulnerability to sudden and incapacitating pain or injury, as well as organ inefficiency and atrophy which includes cardiovascular disease, digestive disorders, migraine headaches, chronic fatigue, and sickness.

Regardless of theory and opinion, the human body is an amazing design. One of the biggest advantages our design affords us is having one spinal column, which allows for three-dimensional movement: twisting; lateral movement; side-to-side movement; and flexion/extension. However, one of the biggest flaws of our design is that we only have one spinal column! If the Locomotor Unit is not balanced and stabilized to hold the one spinal column we have, then there is a large demand placed on the Passenger Unit to try and re-stabilize the body both statically and even more with movement. We would be much better off architecturally if we had two spines. We just would not be able to move very well at all. Our environment and how we currently use our frame, or better yet, do not use our frame, progressively causes an exceptionally large disadvantage over time.

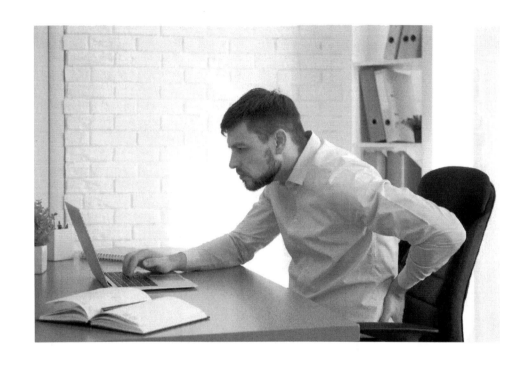

"The profound fact that the human body is designed for movement, exposes the fundamental weakness of our passive western approach to medicine and healing."

~ Patrick Mummy

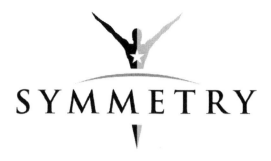

SYMMETRY

THE EFFECTS OF INACTIVITY

Structural alignment provides for the maintenance of homeostasis, active stability, shock absorption, energy conservation, and control and balance. Therefore, a lack of structural alignment provides for the misuse of the systems of our body. It dramatically affects our anatomy, physiology, psychology, and emotional well-being. The resultant symptoms are many. To name of few, this includes dysfunctional hypertrophy (due to chronic overuse), hypotrophy (due to under-use or neuropathy, which is a dysfunction of one or more peripheral nerves, typically causing numbness or weakness), fatigue, rigidity, lack of mobility, instability, depression, insomnia, inability to concentrate, migraine headaches, cardiovascular disease, anxiety, pain, osteoporosis, arthritis, clumsiness, digestive disorders, decreased sex drive, and allergies to name a few.

Misalignment causes fatigue and inflexibility. Both make any type of movement difficult, and more than likely, painful. Pain will further decrease movement and eventually lead to inactivity. The fact that the human body is designed for movement is made more apparent when we examine the flip side of that statement. The human body was not designed for stillness or inactivity. So, when we stand still, we are fighting our natural design and putting our systems under great strain. The average workday for most people today is about 10 hours. Most of that time is usually spent sitting. Sitting is a very inactive state for the body to be in because it disengages the body's primary postural muscle group which is the iliopsoas. Nor are people necessarily active after work. So, for 10 plus hours every day, we fight our natural design and need for movement. We see the consequences of this every day in the Symmetry clinic.

Specific changes that occur to the Locomotor Unit in response to inactivity and improper load bearing are a decrease in oxygen supply due to decreased circulatory system efficiency, a loss of rapid motion and orthostatic tolerance, a decrease of postural sensory signals, and a lessened ability and finite motor acuity because of altered sensory input from both postural and dynamic musculature (Gluckman, 1998).

The time frame for these responses to begin to take place is shown to be 24-72 hours (Vernikos, 2011). The loss of postural cues, due to the deactivation of the antigravity muscles, also begin within this time frame. Since most of our clients have persisted in their postural misalignments for anywhere from two months to 40 years, the serious impact of such findings is quite breathtaking. The fact that Postural Alignment™ Technology can reverse these effects is even more astounding, demonstrating its power and tremendous ability to heal the human body.

The profound fact that the human body is designed for movement exposes the fundamental weakness of our passive western approach to medicine and healing. How can we attempt to help or heal an active entity passively? That would be like giving directions to an English speaker in French. For the body to understand and respond, the approach must be active. This is the power of Postural Alignment Technology™, which asks the body to move in the manner the bones and the muscles tell us the body was designed to move. Hence, we are speaking its language.

Let us take a good look at this language of movement and see where it comes from. Like all languages, it developed over time. So, let us begin with the evolution of the species Homo erectus – the erect man. Millions of years ago man moved back over his hind limbs and stood erect for the first time. No longer would we move on all four limbs. From now on our two hind limbs would be our moving apparatus, and our two front limbs would be free to manipulate the environment and objects in the environment. This new way of being and moving was unique and it provided humans with numerous biomechanical advantages, but it would have large repercussions on our skeletal structure, specifically our spine and balance mechanisms, as well as our psychology, specifically our sense of vulnerability. (Napier, 1967)

Our erect posture demanded that we balance on two feet. This meant that our spine had to shift from one single C-shaped curve supported on either end, to a more cushioning and absorbing S-shaped curve supported on only one end. Standing erect on two feet also shifted our center of gravity further away from the ground, thereby changing the relationship our parts have to each other, as well as their relationships within the body as a whole and with the external environment. How all this made us feel as a species is debatable, yet it is our contention, based on Darwin's Theory of Evolution, that psychologically we are a species based in fear. We fear that we will be destroyed because we know how easily it can happen, given the atavistic awareness of how it was when we were on all fours, when our internal organs were protected by being closer to the Earth's surface and more hidden from possible predators.

The combination of our erect posture and design to move with today's modern, highly technological society has proven disastrous to our health and well-being. We are forced to misuse our skeletal and muscular systems by sitting, wearing clothes, and wearing shoes on our feet. This basically disengages us proprioceptively from our environment, while preserving our ability to survive and provide shelter, food, and protection for ourselves and our family.

Charles Darwin explains the effect of habit, and the use and disuse of parts, as it relates to the evolution of our medical system. We have a built-in inclination for the preservation of favorable individual differences and variations, and for the destruction of those which are

75

injurious and threaten our survival. It would then follow that it would also be instinctual for humans to seek out methods to assist in preservation of these favorable differences and in basic protection. Back in the Ice Age, this instinct led to creating fire, and tools such as the spear, to defend against predators. Nowadays, the threats have changed faces. In place of the saber-toothed tiger and freezing cold, our challenge is inactivity and its intimate link with technology. Our solutions have also changed. We have gone from being primarily active to passive, and because most of our activities are passive, these activities lead us to preserve, rather than eradicate the injurious adaptations that our cultural patterns of inactivity or incorrect activity have subjected us to.

In a nutshell, we mostly sit, and our ancestors did not sit as much as we do today. Sitting deactivates our antigravity muscles. This state of inactivity alters the coordination of responses emitted and received from the central nervous system, which controls all bodily functions. The nervous system has evolved to generate individual behavior that is adaptive within a species' eco niche over a relatively short period of time. Once a young child or teenager has completed the required physical and hormonal development, the body enters a state of homeostasis (Gluckman, 1998). As the child progresses through life and takes on a variety of different postures and forms, this homeostasis is maintained through a system of checks and balances. However, should the body adopt a compromised posture, i.e. one that is lacking the right angle fundamental, over an extended period of time, this system will not be able to return the body back to the original state of homeostasis and skeletal alignment. It will make adaptations and manage the new posture, instead of attempting to change it. Thus, it will formulate a new state of homeostasis. The problem inherent in this process is that this new state is one that is not founded on the right angle fundamental and therefore, not one that allows the body to work effectively with gravity. The result is that gravity has won the war and your body will spend the rest of its time trying to win the battles. This is only if no intervention is sought out and applied to correct the faulty posture.

The body uses two mechanisms to attempt to correct postural misalignment. They are: the stretch sensors deep in the muscles – spindles and the Golgi tendon; and the five righting reflexes, which we previously mentioned. The stretch sensors detect excessive and sudden changes of muscle tension, and the righting reflexes are invoked whenever a body segment deviates from desired postural position. These reflexes attempt to correct the deviation through a signal relayed from a reflex mechanism that causes a muscular contraction (Wikipedia, 2018). There are five righting reflexes:

- optical righting reflex
- body righting reflexes acting on the body
- body righting reflexes acting on the head
- cervical righting reflexes
- labyrinthine righting reflexes

Once the righting reflexes function improperly, the body enters a state of compensated motion. Faulty load bearing and loss of proper postural cues cause compensated motion. Muscular imbalances and the relaying of incorrect neurological signals to incorrect muscles to create movement, typify compensation. The spectrum of imbalance ranges from muscle atrophy to hyper contraction. These are the extremes, and between them are the ranges of weakness or shortness of muscles that affect the segmental body alignment and overall posture (Gluckman, 1998). A person with good overall muscular balance can be realigned through the action of these righting reflexes. However, for those who have weak and dysfunctional muscular patterns that are characterized by an improper response to, or the absence of, a neurological impulse being sent to stimulate deviation correction, neurological reeducation and restoration are needed. Correction and realignment are, therefore, achieved by restoring the proper neurological pathways to the body though the systematic re-education of muscle function, accomplished through our therapeutic exercise program.

In the earlier example of a sprained ankle, systems are functioning to re-attain, in place of maintain, the body's homeostasis. Should the disruption persist for some time, the systems will adapt to become as efficient as possible within this new state. This new state of being will become the new perspective for disruption of homeostasis for that body. Only a furthering of the deviation from the right angle will invoke the righting and stretch sensor reflexes. This is a gradual process of compensation that works to allow compensation to build up and layer itself over the body, cloaking it in an armor of bad habitual posturing.

When we start taking a client through their exercise routines, the body we start with is very rarely the body we will eventually deal with, to move the person eventually out of pain. Taking into consideration everything that you have read up to this point, start thinking about how your own body, and the history of everything you have gone through, relates to the chapters you have read so far. How active have you been throughout your life, and what affect did it, and all the other factors we have discussed, have on your posture? In thinking about this, look at the following pictures. There are four basic postures that most people acquire over their lifetime. Before we move on, determine which of the four basic side postures best fits you and your body. Once you determine what you most look like, ask yourself what experiences in your life may have led to this type of posture.

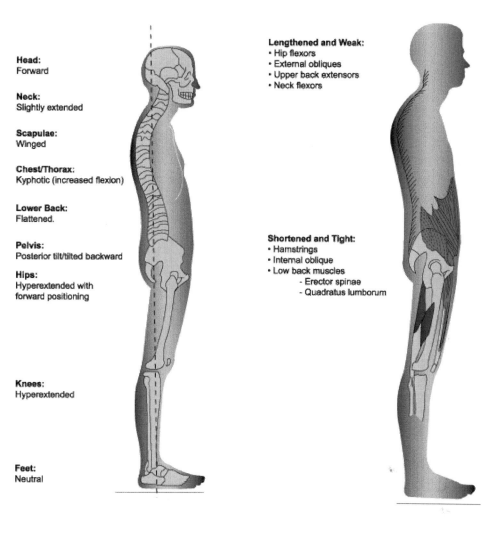

Head:
Forward

Neck:
Slightly extended

Scapulae:
Winged

Chest/Thorax:
Kyphotic (increased flexion)

Lower Back:
Flattened.

Pelvis:
Posterior tilt/tilted backward

Hips:
Hyperextended with
forward positioning

Knees:
Hyperextended

Feet:
Neutral

Lengthened and Weak:
• Hip flexors
• External obliques
• Upper back extensors
• Neck flexors

Shortened and Tight:
• Hamstrings
• Internal oblique
• Low back muscles
    - Erector spinae
    - Quadratus lumborum

Type 1: Kyphosis is associated with an increase curve of the thoracic spine. Along with this, a slightly posterior pelvic tilt is seen along with a reduced lumbar curve and a forward head position. The client will show a hunched over posture with a depressed chest.

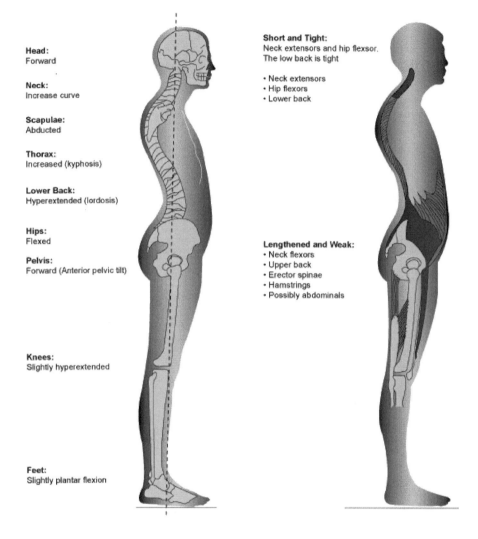

Head:
Forward

Neck:
Increase curve

Scapulae:
Abducted

Thorax:
Increased (kyphosis)

Lower Back:
Hyperextended (lordosis)

Hips:
Flexed

Pelvis:
Forward (Anterior pelvic tilt)

Knees:
Slightly hyperextended

Feet:
Slightly plantar flexion

Short and Tight:
Neck extensors and hip flexsor.
The low back is tight

• Neck extensors
• Hip flexors
• Lower back

Lengthened and Weak:
• Neck flexors
• Upper back
• Erector spinae
• Hamstrings
• Possibly abdominals

Type 2: A sway-back posture can be seen with a neutral or posterior pelvic tilt with the hip almost rolled upward to the front. The client shows a relaxed posture, leaning backwards with the upper body.

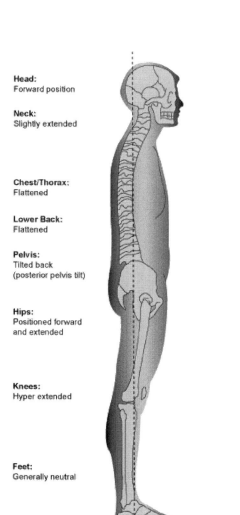

Head:
Forward position

Neck:
Slightly extended

Chest/Thorax:
Flattened

Lower Back:
Flattened

Pelvis:
Tilted back
(posterior pelvis tilt)

Hips:
Positioned forward
and extended

Knees:
Hyper extended

Feet:
Generally neutral

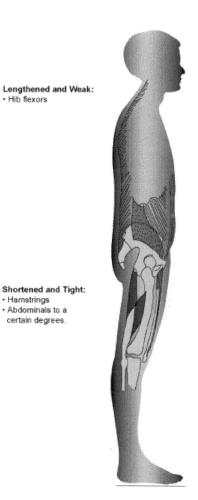

Lengthened and Weak:
• Hib flexors

Shortened and Tight:
• Hamstrings
• Abdominals to a
  certain degrees.

Type 3: A flat back is when little or no lumbar curve is present. There will pretty much always be a posterior pelvic tilt in a neutral position. Occasionally due to the position of the hip it can be difficult to fully straighten the knees when standing.

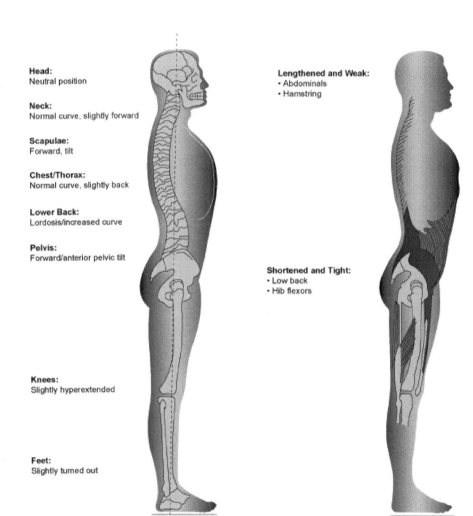

Head:
Neutral position

Neck:
Normal curve, slightly forward

Scapulae:
Forward, tilt

Chest/Thorax:
Normal curve, slightly back

Lower Back:
Lordosis/increased curve

Pelvis:
Forward/anterior pelvic tilt

Knees:
Slightly hyperextended

Feet:
Slightly turned out

Lengthened and Weak:
• Abdominals
• Hamstring

Shortened and Tight:
• Low back
• Hib flexors

Type 4: The Military type posture is more like what correct posture should look like. It is characterized by an increased curve in the lumbar spine of lower back and an anterior pelvic tilt. The client shows a posture in which the chest is pushed forward, shoulders retracted, or pulled back, and load-bearing joints aligned vertically.

82

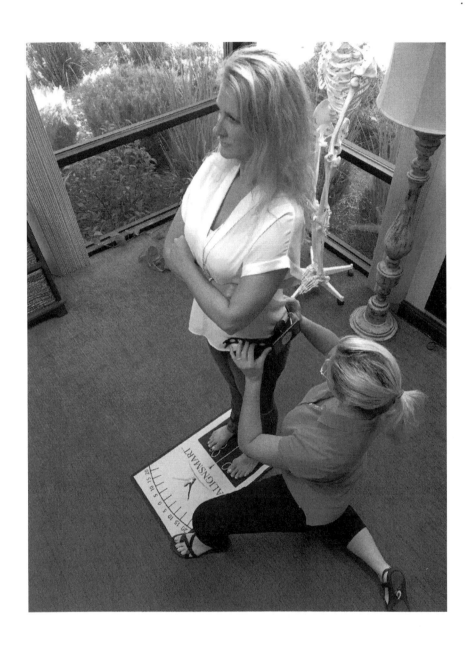

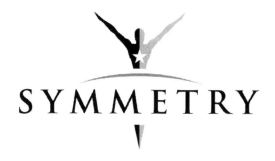

SYMMETRY

POSTURAL ALIGNMENT TECHNOLOGY™

I created Symmetry to fill a void in a system that is more worried about codes and prescriptions than care and long-term results. Symmetry was created to help fill the unanswered questions that so many people have when it comes to their pain. We all have our answers, but we fail to give solutions. When medicine first began, doctors used to make house calls. They had a rapport with their patients. They got to know them intimately and spent the time necessary to make sure their care was beyond adequate. Today, practitioners have to work on volume, or they don't get paid enough to run a business. Practitioners know the limitations of our system and do their best to work within that system. However, I think we can all agree that the system is not as effective as it should be. Why? Because there really isn't an incentive for people to actually get better. Treatments consist primarily of in-clinic care, and our effort is not on what the patient should be doing at home to enhance or continue the healing process. Providers would not get paid for that type of care. As service providers, the issue they face is that if they are not in the office, then they are not getting paid, and therefore become slaves to their job, and eventually it tears them down, and service suffers.

Not so long ago, a new client came into our clinic and began telling me his story that I have heard more than a thousand times in my career. He had a bulged disc for which the doctors recommended surgery and he obliged. Several years later, the same area was affected and to make things worse, he developed herniations in his neck as well. The doctor told him that one had nothing to do with the other. He refused to have another surgery and decided to try other avenues, all of which failed. But the one common theme that he expressed, like so many others, was that he wanted to know what he could do himself that would possibly assist him in becoming healthy and staying healthy. People are starting to change their paradigm about healing, and now, more than ever before, are willing to participate in their own self-care. The internet has helped change this as people are realizing that the success of pain relief is not what we once thought. The stats are there for everyone to see. I remember reading an article in the Los Angeles Times a few years ago where a doctor was asked what his definition of a successful surgery was. His answer was that success was based upon the patient feeling no worse after the surgery. In that same article it was determined that 95% of all back surgeries could be prevented if patients took a more proactive and preventative approach to their bodies, or at least educated and supported in such proactivity.

Symmetry's primary philosophy is based on a client's participation and the support he or she needs to be accountable – all the work to self-heal is continued outside of our office. Our philosophy lies solely on the education of a person to make long-term changes in their everyday habits and have them check in with us consistently. This does two things to ensure success:

1. When our clients get better, they understand that they did the work and view their return to health more as a personal achievement.

2. As a business, we no longer must position our pricing on a per visit basis, but rather as a holistic program that involves both in-office treatment and at-home support. It is our belief that the focus of health care should be 90% education and support and 10% in-office treatment. It is also true that with proper instruction and repeated daily discipline, the body has a natural and amazing capacity to heal itself.

So how does Postural Alignment Technology™ work? As I mentioned previously, the idea behind Symmetry is to give practitioners the tools to be able to better engage with their clients, and help them realize that what they do is making a difference beyond just making them feel better. We have proven that people more than ever want a tangible explanation of why they are feeling better. We have all pledged as practitioners that our number one goal is to help our clients become healthy and pain-free, which ironically, would make them less reliant on us. At first blush, this would seem to decrease revenue. However, what if you could get people better, quickly, while helping them to feel empowered? I can guarantee that you and your client will reap the benefits.

Postural Alignment Technology™ really boils down to simplicity. Geoff Gluckman revolutionized my way of thinking about the body when he talked about the planes of motion, and my enthusiasm was triggered when he described how to assess the body around the planes of motion. When I worked at The Egoscue Method, what we really did was try and assess which muscles were over-engaged and pick exercises that addressed those specific areas. This really is no different than any other therapy. However, because we did not work with planes, it was impossible to assess which tight muscles to work on first. What Geoff explained was that when you are subjectively looking at a body, instead of looking to see what part is out of alignment, look to see from which plane the part of the body is misaligned.

So, if you see an elevated hip for example, the observation is obviously that the hips are not level, but the correct assessment would be that the hip is elevated away from the transverse plane. Why? Because for the pelvis to rotate correctly in the transverse plane, the hips must be level, much like the relationship between a tire and an axel. If there is not a right-angle relationship, then the tire will not rotate correctly. When you look at the body, what you are first recognizing are the imbalances that stand out the most. Understanding what plane these imbalances are deviating away from is crucial to understanding which exercise to choose to correct the specific deviation. I discuss this later. However, what needs to be understood here is that wherever there is an imbalance, the movement within the plane that is deviating away from its natural position will then be compromised.

As I mentioned previously, most practitioners do not take pictures of their clients. This is one of the most important tools for explaining the AlignSmart™ system. Because the entire body is taken under consideration, it is extremely valuable to use a person's pictures to map out their disparities and compensations by showing them the cause behind their pain. It is an exceedingly rare circumstance where a traditional practitioner will take a full body shot and is usually only associated with research. In most cases, an x-ray or MRI will be taken to isolate the painful area and used primarily for explanation. The main purpose for our use of pictures is to make the client aware of the imbalances that they have developed over the years, and to initiate the steps towards an everyday assessment when looking in the mirror each morning.

The problem with most people is the fact that there has been no education about the fundamental principles of the human body as it relates to posture, gravity, and pain. There is no awareness or insight to the predictors of pain because we do not know what to look for, and more importantly, what to expect. Our job is to explain the physics of a person's body in much the same way a structural engineer would explain the physics behind a building or the design of a car. They must be given a tangible comparison to create a clear understanding to the physics behind any structure as it relates to gravity. Pictures are the greatest tools in showing the comparison to what should be and what is in terms of a structural blueprint and how it relates to their current condition. It is the first step to the understanding of the cause of pain. It is commonly referred as a subjective evaluation.

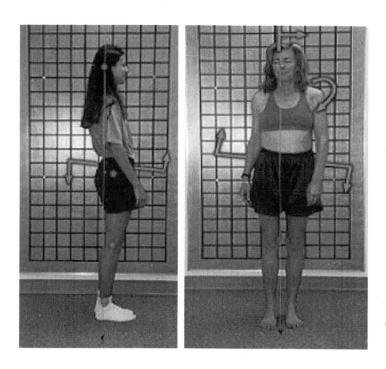

The subjective visual assessment analysis of the human body must begin from a broad perspective. So often the obvious is overlooked because we have tunnel vision in dealing with pain. Therefore, the order of the visual evaluation should be to first find the greatest disparity then continue until you see the least. Remember, you are looking for anything that is skewed from right angles around three-dimensional space first. It is what we refer to as "postural red flags". Have someone take a few pictures of your posture; front, side, and back.

Look at the following list and see if you have any of these visual imbalances:

1. Feet everted, inverted (flat arches or high arches)
2. Hand forward or rounded more than the other
3. Forward rotation of the pelvis (one hip forward of the other)
4. Upper torso rotation (one arm in front more than the other)
5. Scapulae protracted, retracted
6. Scapulae elevated
7. One hip higher than the other
8. More space between one arm and the torso versus the other
9. Knees internal or external or one knee internal and the other external
10. Knees varus or valgus (bow-legged or knock-kneed)
11. Offset of the torso (scoliosis)
12. Offset of the head (lateral tilt)
13. Knee flexion or hyperextension
14. Forward displacement of the pelvis or head from the side view
15. Take notice of muscular asymmetries such as one calf larger than the other, etc.

Now, let us look at the same list above and ask yourself which plane these deviations occur away from. The list below defines this:

1. Feet everted, inverted (flat arches or high arches): **Sagittal**
2. Hand forward or rounded more than the other: **Frontal**
3. Forward rotation of the pelvis (one hip forward of the other): **Frontal**
4. Upper torso rotation (one arm in front more than the other): **Frontal**
5. Scapulae protracted, retracted: **Frontal**
6. Scapulae elevated: **Transverse**

90

7. One hip higher than the other: **Transverse**
8. More space between one arm and the torso versus the other: **Sagittal**
9. Knees medial or external or one knee medial and the other external: **Sagittal**
10. Knees varus or valgus (bow-legged or knock-kneed): **Sagittal**
11. Offset of the torso (scoliosis): **Sagittal**
12. Offset of the head (lateral tilt): **Sagittal**
13. Knee flexion or hyperextension: **Frontal**
14. Forward displacement of the pelvis or head from the side view: **Frontal**

This is the point where we can really impress our clients. With each evaluation you will begin to notice certain patterns that are typical of most individuals. These are what we call rules of thumb. Rules of thumb are derived from the postural red flag analysis and are formally known as righting reflexes. This will be discussed further in the objective evaluation section but should be noted here as well. These rules of thumb correspond with the righting reflexes stated earlier in the book. For example, if one of the obvious disparities you see in your client is a left shoulder elevated, then it can be assumed that the right hip will be elevated. Why? Because most compensations occur from the pelvic level due to the inability to stabilize around the foundation of one's body. If the right hip is elevated, there will be a typical response for the spine to laterally shift away from the elevation. Because the position of the head must be directly in line with the COM in the sagittal plane, a righting response will occur within the left side of the body, thus triggering the trapeziums and corresponding muscles to pull the head back into alignment. This is what I call the Cross-Compensation Effect™. This applies to all other planar compensations as well. Below is a list of typical patterns among normal people when seen for the first time, as well as some general rules for you to learn how to correctly assess and analyze clients:

- Typically, an elevated Iliac Crest (IC) will compensate for the posterior angle of the PSIS-ASIS on the opposite side. However, with athletes it is typically the opposite. The elevated IC is usually the posterior one.
- Shoulder disparities almost always come from pelvic disparities.
- If the IC on one hip is elevated, the opposite side scapulae will usually elevate to compensate.
- If the IC and the scapulae on the same side are both elevated, then the lumbar spine is shifting towards the elevated ilium.
- The body will typically compensate in a way that repositions the head in relationship to the center-point of the pelvis, thus maintaining equilibrium within the body. For instance, if the Greater Trochanter (GT) is displaced forward 4 inches, the upper torso must stay back, and the head will reposition directly vertical to the GT.
- If a hip is elevated, it will laterally shift the spine, and the head will pull back into alignment centered over the pelvis.
- If the pelvis is rotated left to right, then the upper torso will counter-rotate right to left, and the head will rotate back left to right to keep the head balanced within the sagittal plane.
- Thoracic inflexibility corresponds with inflexible hamstrings.
- Valgus knees are more a result of structural compensations, whereas varus knees tend to be more genetic in nature.
- External knees in a sedentary person usually indicate a posterior PSIS-ASIS on the same side.
- External knees on an athlete usually indicate an anterior tilt of the pelvic associated with tight hip flexors.
- Women tend to hyperextend at the knees more than men.
- Medial knees in women usually indicate a posterior PSIS-ASIS angle on the same side and very weak hip flexors.

- Medial knees are indicative of weakness in the frontal and sagittal planes.
- One knee external and one knee neutral or medial indicates a transverse disparity.
- Excess body weight does affect the integrity of a structure but does not restrict one from ridding themselves from pain.
- Runners primarily deviate from the frontal plane.
- Most athletes are typically more misaligned in the transverse plane. This is because most sports are one-side dominant.
- Large inverted/abducted feet and a widened stance are a result of an inability to hold the pelvis in the frontal plane. This reaction occurs as a compensation to widen the support base to decrease the responsibility in the pelvic region.
- Pigeon-toed athletes are faster than duck-footed athletes. This is because our visual assessment of feet that appear pigeon-toed are really aligned. It is not the norm, but from a physics perspective, the more all toes are pointing straight ahead, the greater push-off you can get when running straight ahead. It is called force vectors.
- Everted (pronated) feet indicate a posterior tilt of the same side.
- Ninety-five percent of all normal active children under the age of nine have an anterior tilt of 10 degrees.
- There is a genetic component to some structural abnormalities.
- Form precedes function, in our society.
- Nearly 100% of the population has scoliosis. HOWEVER, the majority have the functional type (not born with it).

Okay, back to the process. I came up with the AlignSmart™ system through a series of trial and error. When I first started Symmetry back in 1997, I was still performing the basic Egoscue Method. Not really knowing what I was doing, but still having decent success. When I went through the Gluckman series, it painted a much clearer picture for me in understanding the dimensional relationships of the body around gravity. But, when I started measuring, it changed the game. By measuring every joint in the body and being able to compare quantitatively how it is positioned against the true skeletal form, it revealed relationships that could not only be explained, but monitored.

In 2003, when I found the programmer for my first software system, I was forced to figure out all the relationships with the measurements and factors I was using during my sessions. Up to that point, I had a rather good understanding of what I was doing, but it still was not as precise as I wanted it to be. I would measure, look at the overall values, start writing down exercises that I knew would correct each disparity, and then try and sequence them appropriately. The problem with this is that I would still tend to pick the same general pool of exercises because the brain (mine in any case) can only hold so much pertinent information at one time. So, the routines ended up looking the same all the time. However, I was still able to monitor the changes in measurements with my clients from session to session, which I found to be a huge advantage regardless of whether my routines were perfect or not.

When we started to create the first software, my wife suggested I write down every factor I used with each client. What I came up with after three months of breaking down, apart, and putting it all together, was a method to sequence corrective exercises that best fit not only the structural deviations of each client, but the emotional/cognitive factors to make sure that they will be consistent in doing the routines in between each appointment. I do not care what healthcare profession you are talking about, there is a sequence to what they do regarding their treatment. However, the biggest issue is that since each evaluation is not quantified, then the practitioner cannot teach the sequence to anyone else due to relying on instinct only. Ultimately, the treatment becomes almost exclusively about diminishing pain or symptoms, and at the end of the day the treatment becomes a series of educated guesses. So, if a client isn't relieved of pain after a few sessions, then that client won't come back, because the practitioner has not given them enough evidence to convince them to stay in treatment, not to mention nothing to give them at home to change habits.

The following are all the factors that are associated with choosing the most effective exercises to correct the current pattern evaluated, and in the best sequence possible. And therefore, I have a patent on this system. Every item is used to generate a specific sequence of corrective exercises. I will talk more about our corrective exercises in a bit because the word exercise is deceiving. Each factor and each measurement combine to create the ultimate sequence to combat the current layer of compensation evaluated. Here are key definitions:

Measurements: It is the crux of our AlignSmart™ Technology. Without the measurements, we have no way to quantify results. Without a way to quantify results, we have no system. Without a system, no one can evidence or replicate the sequence needed to correct a problem. Without a sequence, a practitioner ultimately focuses on ridding you of your pain, which as we have discussed, is the end by-product of your years of compensation. Here is how it works. The body as we have explained works in three planes. You must hold yourself balanced in each plane, using intrinsic muscles, so that you can effectively move within each plane using dynamic muscles. The skeleton, therefore, is strategically designed to support specific muscles that are attached in such a way to optimize this function. We are the only clinic that I know of that does not use muscle testing as our main source of evaluation. What we do is measure 20 bony landmarks which determine, or better yet, map out the static neuromuscular holding pattern around the force of gravity. We do this using our patented Postural Alignment Tool™ and the AlignSmart Technology™ system to quantify these measurements. Remember that ultimately, pain is derived from the inability of muscles to hold and move bones correctly. If we can understand these patterns, then we can generate relational information from the planes that tell us how to correct these patterns.

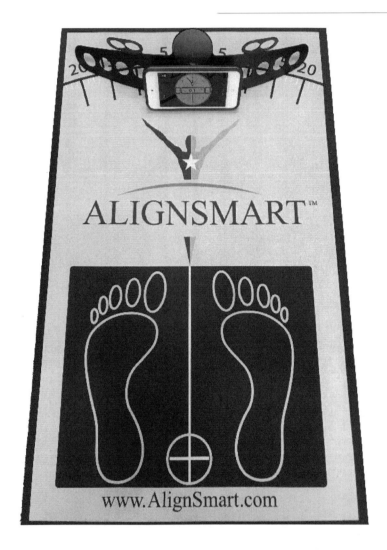

Postural Alignment Kit™ (PAK)

SAGITTAL PLANE

Cervical
Neutral_____
Center to Left S___ M___
Center to Right S___ M___

Thoracic
Neutral_____
Center to Left S___ M___
Center to Right S___ M___

Lumbar
Neutral_____
Center to Left S___ M___
Center to Right S___ M___

Legs-Valgus/Varus
Left
Neutral_____
Valgus S___ M___ L___
Varus S___ M___ L___
Right
Neutral_____
Valgus S___ M___ L___
Varus S___ M___ L___

Knee- Left
External S___ M___ L___
Internal S___ M___ L___
Knee- Right
External S___ M___ L___
Internal S___ M___ L___

Foot- Left
Neutral_____
Everted S___ M___ L___
Inverted S___ M___ L___
Foot- Right
Neutral_____
Everted S___ M___ L___
Inverted S___ M___ L___

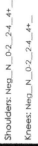

FRONTAL PLANE

Pelvic Rotation
Neutral_____
Left_____
Right_____

Torso Rotation
Neutral_____
Left_____
Right_____

Forward Displacement
Pelvis: N_ 0-2_ 2-4_ 4+_
Head: Neg_ N_ 0-2_ 2-4_ 4-6_ 6+_
Shoulders: Neg_ N_ 0-2_ 2-4_ 4+_
Knees: Neg_ N_ 0-2_ 2-4_ 4+_

Scap Protraction
Left_____
Right_____

Phone #:

TRANSVERSE PLANE

PSIS-ASIS
Left_____
Right_____

Iliac Crest
Neutral_____
Left_____
Right_____

Scapuale Elevation
Neutral_____
Left_____
Right_____

FACTORS

ABILITY
Low
Medium
High

AVAILABILITY
Low
Medium
High

DOD
Low
Medium
High

RAMPING
Supine
Prone
Buddhas Pose
Kneeling
Sitting
Standing

FLEXIBILITY

Thoracic
Low
Medium
High

Groin
Low
Medium
High

Hamstrings
Low
Medium
High

SYMPTOMS
(scale 1-10)
1)
2)
3)
4)

NAME:

EMAIL:

Ability to Follow Directions: The ability of a client refers to the kinesthetic awareness a person displays as it pertains to being able to follow directions with the exercises suggested. If a client has an Average Ability to follow directions, this means that they more than likely do not have the awareness to perform complex exercises correctly and will more than likely perform it incorrectly at home. Above Average Ability means that they do have the ability to follow directions, complex or not.

Degree of Difficulty (DOD): This refers to how hard you want the client to work in a routine. A Low DOD means that most exercises will be passive, whereas a high DOD means that most exercises will require a high-level of effort or work. A lot of this, however, is determined by the symptoms of a client as well. Most of the initial exercises suggested are isometric in nature due to the high level of correction they provide.

Ending Position: This factor refers to the position in which the client finishes their routine. For example, if you choose supine, then all the exercises will be on the floor, on the back. As I previously stated, it literally takes on average one year to get from the floor to standing from the time we are born. This is the ramping process that the brain must develop around to connect the neuromuscular dots. When a client comes in for each appointment, we must determine if they indeed can get to a standing position without the overall compensation correction being negatively affected. I know this sounds a bit funny, because most people can stand; however, if we add more and more levers around gravity, and the body cannot handle the load due to the amount of compensation accrued over the years, then the body will default back to its known or remembered holding patterns, which will render the sequence null and void. This is one of my biggest criticisms of most therapies or training sessions. Most people cannot hold their own body weight correctly around gravity, so when you try and treat or train the body in a dysfunctional position, standing being the most prevalent, all you are doing is strengthening this dysfunction. Thus, no new patterns are engrained.

Flexibility: There are three main areas for flexibility: Thoracic, Groin, and Hamstring. This is an overall assessment of a client's flexibility which will ultimately determine which exercise they can perform or not. Check out the steps below and assess your own flexibility.

1. **Thoracic**

    a. Sit on a chair with your knees bent at 90 degrees.

    b. Interlace your hands pushing your palms away. While locking your elbows, raise your arms overhead and behind your head as far as possible without leaning backwards.

    c. Assess your flexibility in three categories: Low, Medium, or High.

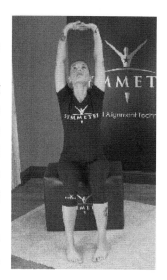

- Low: You have an extremely difficult time locking your arms and pulling them to the front of your face.
- Medium: You have a reasonable ability to pull your arms back and can get your arms parallel to your head.
- High: You have no problem pulling your arms behind your head.

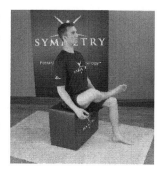

2. **Groin**

    a. Sit on a chair with your knees bent at 90 degrees.

99

b. Place an ankle to the opposite knee (both sides). The leg that has the lowest flexibility is the one you record.

- Low: You have an extremely difficult time pushing your knee away and have a hard time even getting the ankle to the knee.
- Medium: You have a reasonable ability to push your knee away.
- High: You have no problem pushing your knee away.

3. **Hamstrings**

a. Stand with your feet hip width apart.

b. While keeping your legs locked, slowly bend at the waist and try and touch your toes.

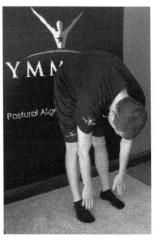

- Low: Client has an extremely difficult time bending down and can barely reach their knees.
- Medium: Client has a reasonable ability to reach past their knees and to their ankles.
- High: Client has no problem touching their toes or the floor.

Area of Concern: Remember, we really are not dealing with symptoms; we are dealing with the cause of the symptoms. However, if someone has been injured by a contact accident and they are in acute pain, this program is probably inappropriate at this juncture and may not be suitable until one has stabilized the injured area. Remember, we are focusing on getting rid of the pain by understanding how to treat the cause. Just by evaluating your client correctly, you will more than likely be able to accurately guess where your client's discomfort is located. However, we still need to understand where and what the symptoms are so that we do not exacerbate them and can at least monitor the pain throughout the course of treatment. So, when an area is chosen in the software, all exercises contraindicated for this area will not be picked in the sequence.

When I have a new client in front of me, I literally tell them that if the main objective in coming to our office is to get rid of pain, then they are in the wrong clinic. Our main objective is putting his or her body back into proper form, thus proper function, and the result will be a decrease or ridding of his or her issues. It is that simple. Our method of alignment explains how the body is changing and how we must unravel years of compensation first before we can strengthen them completely. We coach our clients through the entire process. Clients stick with us for the first three-month corrective phase of the program and finally get out of pain due to the complexity of their compensation patterns. But they stick with us because we can show them where their bodies were, where they are now, and where we know they will go.

It is physics, and if we have a proactive client, we know we have someone that will beat their years of chronic pain and dysfunction. It just takes time, education, commitment, and motivation. Most therapies do not work simply because people do not spend enough time in the process to allow the body to heal! So, if you were to have evidence that you were going in the right direction, I certainly know that you would be more willing to stay engaged in the process. Yes, some of our clients are so badly compensated that they need more than the first three months to heal, but we stay with them until they do. This should be the healthcare model in which we all engage and participate.

You are probably asking, "How do I measure myself?" The answer is you cannot! Not effectively anyway. This is the problem with self-help books. They can only help you to a certain degree, and then they become ineffective because you are too unique as an individual, with too many differences. Grouping everyone in the same manner neglects major factors that should determine your individual treatments. Again, this is my main criticism of yoga classes or any other group classes. If you want to be measured, give us a call and we will locate a Symmetry AlignSmart™ Practitioner near you!

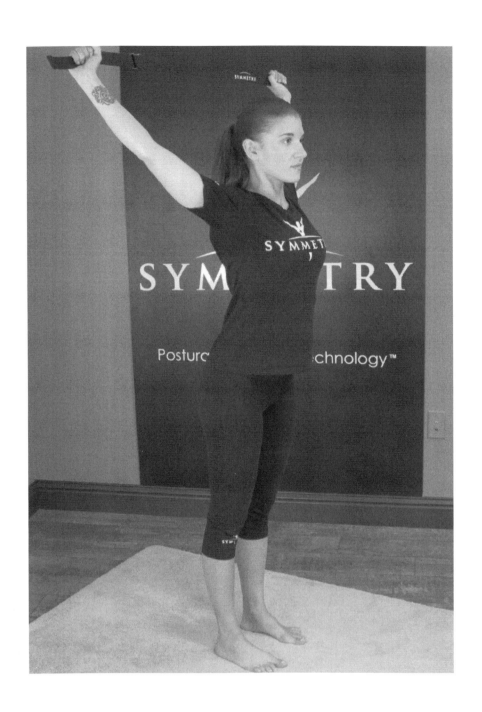

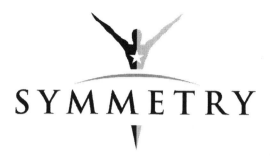

SYMMETRY

THE EXERCISES

This is where the rubber meets the road. In today's physical health world there are many philosophies behind getting people strong and out of pain. I hear almost daily where a new client will come in and tell me that their doctor or healthcare provider has strongly suggested that they increase their core workout to help strengthen their back. In typical rehab treatments, most of the exercises prescribed are focused on the pain area itself. Another is, "I was told to get back in the gym and start strength training". At Symmetry, we do not encourage these practices initially. As we explained previously, if your frame is bent, it does not matter what car you drive or what you 'fix', you are still out of alignment. I mentioned in the first chapter that going into my senior year at SDSU I went from bench pressing 200 pounds to 300 pounds in a matter of months. What I didn't explain to you was that every time I went into the weight room, my left hip angle was posterior, my right ilium was elevated, my pelvis was rotated left to right, and my right shoulder was very protracted and elevated. These were just some of my issues, but what I was not told was that I had to prepare my structural body before any of my activities. I was told to build my core strength and to stretch as much as I could. Well, I am here to tell you that I did both to the extreme. But it was not too soon into my senior year that I quickly realized that every time I stretched before a game, I would get injured.

In 2006, I had the opportunity to follow Az Hakim when he re-signed with the Detroit Lions. He introduced me to their strength and conditioning Coach Bert Hill. I remember Bert asking me once what I thought about his linemen stretching before a game or practice. I told him I did not like it the way it is typically approached. He agreed, stating many references to research that indicated that stretching before activity caused more injuries. So, he told me that they did more warm-up drills than traditional stretching. I did not go into my theories with him at the time, but if I had I would have given the opinion that he was wrong. You see, I am not against stretching per se, I am against stretching in and of itself, by itself. What I mean by this is that I found out half-way through my senior season that when I did concentrate on stretching prior to a game, I usually had some type of injury during the game. So, I too, began just performing some general warm-up drills, such as wind-sprints, to loosen up my body. But stretching is not the problem.

Knowing what I know now, I realize that what people do when they just concentrate on stretching, is to lengthen a tight muscle. But when you understand physics and compensation patterns, what you will end up realizing yourself, is that when you stretch out your tight muscles, you are in fact stretching out the muscles that your brain has recruited to help stabilize an imbalanced frame. Each week at our clinic, I get a client that will come in and tell me that they had a bad reaction to a massage or adjustment. Same thing. If you understand the main component of any typical passive treatment model such as massage, acupuncture or chiropractic, you are dealing with a passive client lying on a table and getting rubbed, needled, or adjusted. The common denominator is a release occurs, which will feel exceptionally good initially. But quite soon after, your muscular default pattern will reengage because you did nothing to strengthen the change that just occurred. So, when you release tight muscles and do not strengthen the imbalance that caused the tightness in the first place, your brain says, no! Then, pulls you back into protection mode.

So, the type of exercises used to correct misalignments is extremely important when trying to figure out how to rid someone of pain. When people ask what type of exercises we use at Symmetry, we usually explain that our system is most like scientific yoga, in a sense. Yoga primarily uses isometric exercises, which are the best form of exercises to change posture, but there is no measuring, and therefore, everyone goes through the same sequence. We get a lot of clients who come in injured from performing yoga. However, if we taught yoga instructors the AlignSmart™ system, it would be a game changer. In the meantime, let us dive deeper into the different types of exercises used at Symmetry. There are four categories of exercises used, each type for a specific purpose.

1. **Passive**: a passive exercise is one that has _no work_ associated with it. It is typically a releasing exercise or a resting exercise such as the Static Floor or Wall Groin Stretch. This would be considered a static stretching exercise where the body is positioned on the floor using multiple reference points to allow the weight of the body to act upon a joint or joints. Staying in this passive position long enough allows for the brain to disengage due to no work being done, and for compensated muscle groups to _let go_, allowing for temporary relief.

2. **Isometric**: an isometric exercise is one that provides *work without movement* and describes most of the Symmetry postures. These exercises can include more isometric stretching (Piriformis Crossovers) or strengthening (Wall Sits). _Isometric exercises_ are considered the most appropriate for changing postural misalignment because these most directly influence the intrinsic musculature due to intrinsic muscles not changing length with external force. Therefore, to move the body dynamically will not change the postural position of the body but only enhance the

107

compensation patterns already developed. Here are the benefits of isometric training (breakingmuscle.com):

- One of the main benefits of isometric training *is that the body can activate nearly all the available motor units – something that is usually exceedingly difficult to do.* Back in the 1950s, researchers Hettinger and Muller found a single daily effort of two-thirds of a person's maximum effort, exerted for six seconds at a time for ten weeks, increased strength about 5% per week. Clark and associates demonstrated static strength continued to increase even after the conclusion of a five-week program of isometric exercises.

- Another benefit of isometric training is simply the amount of time spent performing an exercise. Consider an exercise like the bench press. It may take one to two seconds to perform with each joint angle only being trained for short periods of time. In contrast, an exercise that mimics the bench press, like a press against pins at the sticking point of the lift, may be performed for several seconds. *In other words, if you have a problem at a joint angle in a lift, you can do targeted isometrics to quickly overcome your problems.*

- Given that you can perform isometrics with little equipment and a relatively short timeframe, you would think they would be far more popular in the training world. So why aren't they mainstream? For starters, there is no denying the *commercial aspect*. With isometrics, there is no valuable equipment to sell. Secondly, there has been some selective use of the science involved in isometric research.

- Like all good training methods, *you need to know how and when to apply isometrics, and how to overcome whatever shortfalls it has.* Every system has holes in it, but our job is to explain to you how to overcome it. Potential decreases in muscle elasticity and speed of movement are easy to overcome with the use of relaxation and stretching methods such as we use in Symmetry.

- Research has shown that because of the reduced blood flow during prolonged muscle tension, numerous growth factors remain in the muscle tissue longer and stimulate muscle growth. Doing a higher number of contractions increases strength, while holding contractions longer increases muscle mass.

- Convenient style of training at any place and at almost any time. Isometric exercises can provide a source of strength training at any place and whenever you feel like it. While there is some equipment that you may find useful for isometric exercises at the gym, you can perform these exercises without any equipment at all, making it very convenient while helping you maintain your fitness goals.

- May be helpful to someone who is healing from an injury. Isometric exercises provide a source of strength training without the impact that more complex exercises may require. For example, if you have a shoulder injury, a physical therapist may recommend some isometric exercises that stabilize the shoulder and maintain strength in that area so that the recovery is faster.

- May help lower blood pressure. The Mayo Clinic notes that a recent study has shown that isometric exercises may also help *naturally lower your blood pressure* since exercising at higher intensities can cause a dramatic increase in your blood pressure, specifically during the activity. Regardless, it is important to check with your doctor before beginning isometric exercises if you have high blood pressure or any heart problems. Also, please note that isometric exercise can also increase blood pressure during performance; however, a regular exercise program generally helps reduce blood pressure. A study conducted by the Division of Cardiology at University Health Network in Toronto, Canada suggests that isometric exercise training in young and old participants may produce reductions in blood pressure. In this case, isometric exercise training protocols typically consisted of four sets of two-minute handgrip or leg contractions sustained at 20–50 percent of maximal voluntary contraction, with each set separated by a rest period of one to four minutes. Training was usually completed three to five times per week for four to 10 weeks. Improvements in the regulation of heart rate and blood pressure have been reported. Some key things to remember - never hold your breath or strain during any training exercise as this may cause a dangerous rise in blood pressure.

- Relieve depression. American physician and cardiologist, Dr. Paul Dudley White, a prominent advocate of preventive medicine, states that, "Healthy exercise is valuable not only for the maintenance of good physiologic function of the body, but also mental clarity, and a feeling of good health". It has long been known that exercise serves as a *natural remedy for depression* in all ages, regarding how they feel about themselves. Self-concept denotes a set of thoughts held by oneself and about one's self in mental, emotional, and physical realms. Self-esteem refers to the individual's evaluation of his or her self-concept, and self-efficacy is like self-confidence in that self-efficacy is a level of certainty that one can perform a task or behavior.

3. **Active Isometric (Isotonic):** an active isometric exercise is one that *provides specific movement of a joint or joints off an isometric holding position* and does not displace the body over a measurable distance. For example, Hip Rotations, Shoulder Rotations, and Inverted Rotations are examples of Transverse Plane active isometric exercises. These exercises are also focused on correcting misalignment, but also add a strengthening component due to the movement. These exercises use multiple reference points to position the body at right angles to recruit a bilateral engagement or specific joint movement.

4. **Dynamic:** dynamic exercises displace the body over a measurable distance and involve more than one lever. They are designed to strengthen the dynamic muscles to secure an aligned posture. Examples of this would be cross-training, weightlifting, plyometrics, etc.

In summary, the cerebellum, a small part of our lower brain in the back of the head, plays a vital role in coordinating muscles, controlling many reflexes, and keeping us erect in the earth's gravitational field. Recent research demonstrates that the cerebellum contributes to the control of all brain functions, especially cognition and behavior, and may be just as great as its control over motor. The cerebellum receives a great portion of its input from the receptors embedded in the joints and muscles. Although humans are not constantly moving, there is continuous stimulation to the cerebellum from the mechanoreceptors in the joints and muscles, due to the constant load on these structures as a result of gravity. Gravity is thus responsible for providing a source of constant stimuli to our brain.

If the joints and muscles of the body, especially the spinal joints, which receive the majority of the force in the upright posture of humans, are moving correctly, then there is an optimum amount of mechanoreceptor stimulation to the cerebellum and brain. This results in an appropriate control of the postural muscles. The postural muscles then have increased endurance, allowing them to hold an individual upright for long periods of time. If an individual has altered biomechanics/movement of a joint, then he or she may have a decreased amount of mechanoreceptor stimulation to the brain and, in turn, have decreased stimulation to the postural muscles. This could result in a decreased efficiency of these muscles, leading to the question which often arises: What is the best way to improve or maintain postural integrity?

Although exercise of the back muscles is extremely important in this process, many of these back muscles are non-consciously, reflexogenically, controlled by the cerebellum; therefore, exercise has a minimal effect. The deepest muscles throughout the spine (together called the intrinsic layer) extend from one vertebra to the next, making them completely dependent on joint motion and reflexive control from the cerebellum. Therefore, isometric exercises are the most effective in retraining posture because they are most associated with the brain. Another aspect, which I mentioned in the last chapter, was about the ramping factor of a routine. We discussed the amount of time it takes for the average child to get on their feet from birth. The main goal of writing a routine is to progressively ramp a client to the point of standing. With this in mind, we are taking into consideration the number of levers used from start to finish, the goal being to tie the levers as neurologically coordinated as possible so that the brain can understand how to re-pattern one's alignment for a long-term hold. The following list of positions from least number of levers to the most is necessary to understand how to ramp a routine properly:

1. Lying- the supine position (on your back)
2. Prone-the prone position (on your stomach)
3. Elbows and knees
4. Hands and Knees
5. Sitting on the floor
6. Kneeling- a position of one on their knees only
7. Sitting on a chair
8. Standing

With these positions in mind it is especially important to understand that there is a varied degree of difficulty based on the movement or work being done in each position. The following pictures describes the basic positions from which all Symmetry corrective postures are derived.

Supine-Static Floor: This is the most basic position to give a client. The Static Floor position provides the body with the most stability because it has the most reference points to support the entire body in a horizontal position, thus 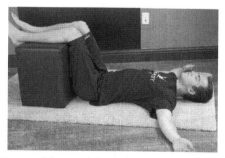 allowing the brain to relax fully. From this position there are many exercises that can be performed in all three planes due to the overall stability it provides. The key in this position is to have the hips and knees bent at a 90-degree angle so that the spine is neutral. If a person's legs are too long, then a pillow or blanket can be added on top of the chair for better positioning. Conversely, if a person's legs are too short, a different chair or block should be used.

Supine- Bent Legs: This position requires the knees to be bent and feet hip-width. The best way to get into this position is to start with your feet together in the midline of the body, then separate your heels out wide keeping your toes 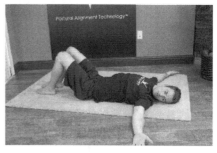 together, and then slightly separate your feet apart so that you feel slightly pigeon-toed. This places your feet and knees in the correct starting position, with your legs parallel. From here there are a multitude of exercises that can be performed in all three planes, but this is the best starting position. This position lessens the amount of support for the legs, which makes the work a little harder due to the natural arch induced in the low back.

Supine-Feet on Wall: This position requires your feet to be on the wall with your hips and knees bent at a 90-degree angle. Again, place your feet hip-width, using the same positioning as described in the bent-leg description. From this 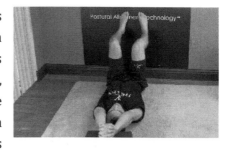 position, a multitude of exercises can be performed in all three planes. The key with this position is to make sure the feet stay in the same position. With the feet on the wall, this activates the hip flexors as the legs are required to perform more work holding the feet on the wall.

Supine-Inverted Wall: This position requires your legs to be all the way up against the wall, with your torso straight out from the wall, legs hip-width apart. With your legs straight up, you have increased the length of the levers which makes this position 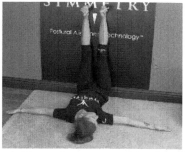 harder than the previous three described. From here a multitude of exercises can be performed in all three planes. If you need, back your tailbone away from the wall in order to keep your tailbone on the floor.

Prone Position: This position is where the spine comes off the floor for the first time. Due to being suspended on the floor, the spine will naturally increase in extension in this position. From here, there are a multitude of 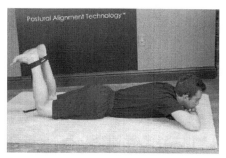 exercises in all three planes that can be performed, from extremely easy to extremely difficult. With each exercise, make sure the directions are being followed closely as there are a variety of positional changes that can occur from this starting position.

Elbows and Knees: This position is where the spine and torso are suspended off the floor, in which the pelvis and the shoulder girdle are required to stabilize the spine. In most of the exercises in this position, the shoulder blades are 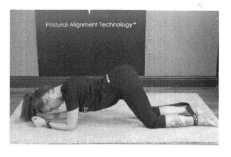 required to collapse as well as the low back, to provide a stretch or traction in the spine to help provide extension between vertebrae. The work required in this position is now increased as this position starts

115

to tie the connection between the locomotor unit and the passenger unit.

Hands and Knees: This position emulates the crawling stage of development in our first year of life. This is where the hip flexors begin to recognize their function, bridging the gap of stability from the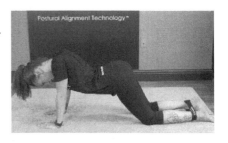
Locomotor Unit to the Passenger Unit. This position also requires extension in the low to mid back to provide length in a body that is usually compressed due to compensation. The work in this position becomes more difficult due to the extending of the arm levers but provides a good stability position for correction in all three planes.

Sitting-Floor: The next stage of development is sitting on the floor. There are a variety of sitting-floor positions, so the directions will vary depending on the exercise and the plane being addressed. The key here is that this is where the spine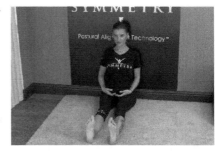
begins to transition to a vertical loadbearing position, but off a flexed pelvis. It starts the connection from the Locomotor Unit to the Passenger
Unit for the ability of the entire body to stand and provides a great transitional setting for more core strength work.

Kneeling: The kneeling position is now where the Passenger Unit and the Locomotor Unit begin to balance with each other around the force of gravity. With balancing the pelvis on top of the femurs only, this position provides great stability and extension of the hips and the spine. It begins the 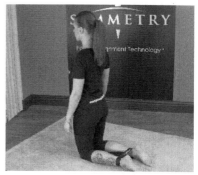 connection of the intrinsic patterning between the legs, pelvis, and spine to be able to stand correctly around the planes of motion. Make sure the knees are hip width apart depending on the exercise, but a variety of positions can be obtained for both correction and strength.

Sitting: The sitting position is environmentally what has caused our society to lose its structural integrity. But with this position, it helps to focus on the passenger unit extending on top of the pelvis to strengthen the tie from legs as the origin and the spine as the insertion point. Done properly, this position helps to strengthen the 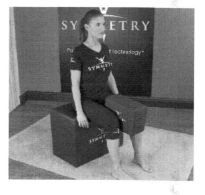 transition to standing. Make sure the knees are at 90-degrees, feet hip-width in order to provide the maximum leverage for the hip flexors and back muscles to engage properly. What is emphasized in this position is sitting tall by rolling the pelvis forward, allowing the torso to extend up, shoulders retracted, and chin down. This helps to train the spine to be in its proper vertical position.

Standing: Standing and moving on two legs is the inherent design and function of our bodies. Ultimately our goal is to train the body to statically hold itself as extended and balanced three-dimensionally as possible for it to move effectively around gravity. Therefore, when performing exercises in this position, it is vital that the directions are followed closely as this position is also where the body can compensate the most due to all the levers being used around gravity. There are very many exercises that can be given in this position in all three planes, mostly for strengthening purposes.

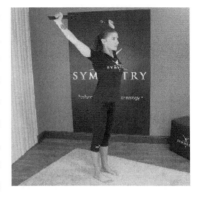

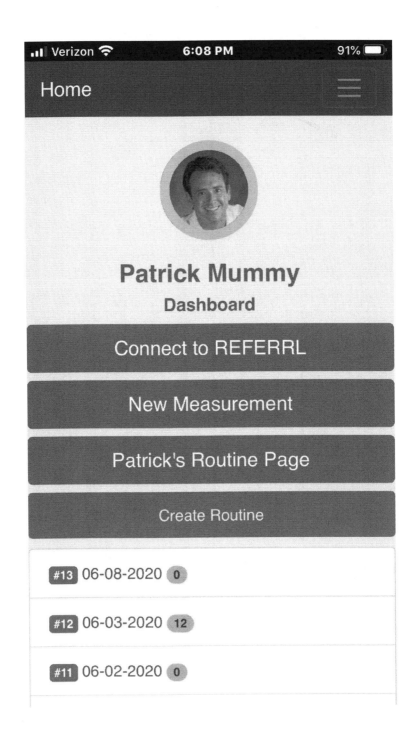

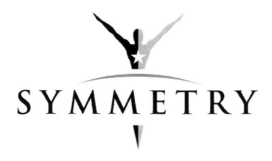

SYMMETRY

THE ALIGNSMART™ TECHNOLOGY

I was awarded a patent for this system in 2007. We applied for it in 2003. My advice to you if you are seeking one, start now, and wait impatiently! This system is based on six main steps:

1. Measure the client/you.
2. Label the factors for each client (as stated in the last chapter).
3. Generate a report.
4. Create a sequence.
5. Take client/you through the routine.
6. Feel great!

Being that we have already discussed the first two steps, let us talk more about step three. It is one thing to assess a client. It is another to quantify a system with measurements. I remember when I was in San Diego, I was able to set up a meeting with the top five Physical Therapists (PT) from Sharp Rees-Stealy, one of the main medical groups there. As I do with most of my presentations, I asked them if any one of them had any chronic pain. Three out of the five said they did. One volunteered who said he had a chronic shoulder problem. While facing away with his shirt off, I asked the remaining PTs to tell me which shoulder looked elevated. They correctly chose the right, because subjectively, it was obviously higher than the left. I then took my

Palpation Meter, which is the tool I had at the time, and proceeded to measure the inferior borders of both scapulae, of which it read seven degrees high on the right side. I then explained that this is an objective way of taking out the "guess work" from typical postural analysis. I then asked them what they thought his pelvis was doing. They looked at me and said, "I'm not sure what you mean?"

I then went into my discussion of physics- Newton's Third Law, and the righting reflex. I explained that the odds were that his left ilium was elevated. I then took my fingers and palpated the crest of his pelvis, of which you could clearly see that his left hip was elevated. I then measured it, and it read 7 degrees elevated on the left hip. I turned around fully expecting to see looks of amazement, but rather was asked, "How accurate is that device?" You see, in the mainstream medical institution, practitioners are not taught physics as it relates to the human body, nor are they taught to measure posture. In the PT world, measuring joint flexibility is about the extent of any measuring performed, and a good PT will palpate landmarks to explain that certain joints might be despaired, but there is no system of explaining why you might be out of alignment and moreover, how to get back into alignment. Regardless of whether anyone thinks my system is inaccurate or scientifically sub-par, the industry should have a similar software program where patients can view their specific rehab exercise videos and report back to their practitioner consistently with support, in order to promote compliance.

The answer is very simple- our medical model does not incentivize the patient to change habits at home. Practitioners get paid to treat symptoms, label a code for that treatment, and then bill your insurance. They do not get paid for changing your habits at home; they only get paid for office visits. I had a client who recently had surgery on her shoulder to clear out some calcium deposits, and after was prescribed PT. The PT explained that they had to manipulate the insurance companies because the insurance companies only give them a specific amount of treatments per ailment. He expressed that if she wanted to continue working on the same area, she would have to go back to the doctor for a different diagnosis, then come back to him so that he could continue working on her shoulder. The medical system the way it currently operates does not work well enough.

Okay, so, quantifying a system goes beyond just measuring. You must know how to interpret the measurements, which is what makes a system a system. So, how did I come up with the AlignSmart™ system? It started with the very first software programmer I hired back in 2002. We had him go through the Symmetry program as if he was a typical client, so that he could experience the system personally. From this experience, the main thing he told me was that everything in code is just mathematical equations or numbers. So, I had to create an algorithm that explained the relationships between the planes of motion, the measurements within each plane, and the factors associated as numerical values. And that is what I did. What I discovered is that the number of measurements in the transverse plane is less than the frontal plane, which is less than the number of measurements in the sagittal plane. This is because we are primarily sagittal-moving beings as this is the plane in which we primarily move.

If you look at dynamic training, the majority of movements are linear or flexion/extension due to the fact that this is the easiest and most effective way of moving our body from point A to point B. Alas, I keep talking about structural holding patterns. So, mathematically, if you were to develop a weighted system so that you could quantify the planar relationships, then you would have a way to figure out what disparity is the most important in the process of correcting intrinsic disparities. Let us take most postural assessment programs. These are almost entirely composed of *seeing the disparity*, and not *measuring the disparity*. Again, this is a generic way of evaluating the body, which results in generic treatments. When you place the body in planar categories and then weigh the planar categories, it becomes noticeably clear as to what needs to be corrected first. The sequence is the key to success. If you cannot explain objectively why you are treating someone in the sequence you perform, then you cannot expect to ever replicate yourself. From this mentality, and after analyzing the planar relationships and weighting the categories appropriately, I created what I call the Severity-Disparity Chart™.

This chart (which is part of the propriety information in our patent), explains exactly how I weighted each measurement within each plane, and then how it relates from plane to plane. Ultimately, this is where a sequence is derived, but for our purposes here, it is important for you to know that if you do not have values assigned in the proper algorithm, then it is impossible to really know where to start your treatment. This is where I always got lost when I was at the Egoscue Method. There were no manuals or equations to guide me to know where to start and where to end. At the end of the day, it was just a series of guesses and hope that a client responded positively to the exercises.

What I can tell you is that if you look at the ratio between the planes, there is basically a 1:2:3 relationship between the Transverse, Frontal, and Sagittal planes, and the measurements involved. The Transverse plane, being the only horizontal plane, will be the most sensitive to any type of disparity due to the attachments around this plane, and therefore is weighted more heavily in the evaluation process. It is also the most compensated plane because most people are one-side dominant. So, when a person rotates, it is usually to one side primarily, thus promoting over-development of that side. That was me in my 16 years of playing baseball. But it can be as simple as repetitively rotating to one side at your desk sitting in front of your computer. Depending on the patterns developed over the years, this is the reason why most people come into our office with large PSIS-ASIS disparities.

However, you cannot see this measurement! The only way you can understand that there is such a disparity is if you know what you are looking for, which in most cases is a reaction to this disparity. Pelvic rotation, an elevated ilium, knee rotation, or spinal offsets; these are all results of a PSIS-ASIS disparity. At the end of the day, even if you do know what you are looking for, you do not know to what degree the disparity occurs, and whether or not it needs to be addressed initially. What I do know is that no therapy can measure this or any of the other landmarks, thus making the mistake of treating the by-product result, which is usually the site of pain. In our system, I can tell you that almost all clients who come in initially are more despaired in the transverse plane, which should be addressed initially before anything else.

In my opinion, the mistake that most clinical therapists make is addressing a patient's issues with sagittal plane exercises first (flexion/extension). Let me give you an example. In the foreword, Az mentioned my prediction of Deuce McAllister, the running back for the Saints who ended up injuring his knee. What he did not mention is that towards the end of the season, I got a chance to meet Deuce and was able to discuss my philosophy about his knee injury. He told me that he had been in Florida with the team's top physical therapist rehabbing his knee for two months. But when I measured him, I found that his right hip was elevated eight degrees, anteriorly tilted 14 degrees, and his left hip was posteriorly rotated five degrees. The imbalance in his pelvis was so blatant, and so obvious to me why his right knee gave out. But he had been rehabbing for two months on his knee only, and not the cause behind it!

As I reviewed his report, I explained that his opposite hip was so posterior that it was causing his right hip to take on most of the compensation, leading his knee to externally rotate on the same side. The side he injured and had surgery work performed. You cannot just simply treat an area of pain without understanding the source from which it emanates. This is how traditional therapy works. Most knee rehab work is done in the Sagittal plane flexion/extension. However, if the problem originates from the PSIS-ASIS, then this must be corrected with rotational exercises first before you can even think about rehabbing the knee. Treatment protocols are based on injuries and not the cause of injury. So, you see, sequence matters. It matters a lot because if you are treating the body in the wrong order, then the default pattern of compensation will always win. This is also why adjustments rarely hold. But with a properly sequenced routine, *in conjunction with any treatment*, the body will recover faster than you can imagine!

So, let us talk about the system itself. I have spent over 25 years developing a system that not only quantifies the why statements behind the cause of pain, but also allows for proper support, education, and motivation to engender compliance. When I first started Symmetry back in 1997, it was not more than a few years later where I had a conversation with an orthopedic surgeon I knew. I remember specifically explaining Symmetry and what I had created, the philosophy, and how it helped clients manage and solve their issues by giving them a plan at home to follow. His response was the same as almost every licensed healthcare professional I have come across thereafter. He exclaimed, "Patrick, this sounds like a great program, but people are innately lazy and don't want to be held responsible for changing or treating themselves".

This paradigm is why I have never quit Symmetry and have spent years trying to perfect a system that can change habits. To reemphasize what I have said previously in this book, the only way one is going to resolve long-term issues is to learn how to create new habits that allow the body to make the changes needed to become healthy again. Taking responsibility of one's own health is an extremely hard task in and of itself. But by one's self without the help or support of a system, it can be extremely daunting and usually ends up losing out to original habits—bad habits. What I have observed in my career over time, is that people are fed up with being in pain, and not receiving the education and support necessary from our healthcare system to make a real difference. We pay an extremely high price in our monthly healthcare insurance premiums to simply receive Band-Aid care, shifting from one treatment to another, with no long-term results. According to medicinenet.com, a recent study published in the Journal of Pain, found average adults suffering from moderate pain paid nearly $9,000 per year for health care costs. The healthcare system is broken.

In any case, the process of using and accessing The AlignSmart Technology™, is a more detailed discussion, and for our purposes here, I will give you a quick look into how it works and how it is used. For more options to get involved with our program, whether you are a practitioner wanting to augment your own practice, or a client who is frustrated with the system, a more in-depth explanation of these options and processes are described in more detail in the *Training and Certification* chapter.

AlignSmart™ Technology for the Practitioner

As I have mention previously, the technology we have created both serves the practitioner and the client. For the practitioner, the software is where all the data is entered, and routines created. The process is rather easy, but inputting the data is necessary in the education and treatment of the client. Once a practitioner has pulled up the client's dashboard, a *New Measurement* tab is selected, and this is where the measurements are entered. From here, a report is generated that explains the compensation patterns that are showing and how it relates to the pain the client may be experiencing. The software automatically weighs each measurement within each plane and comes up with a total score at the top of each plane reflecting the severity of compensation showing in each plane. The score for each planar measurement has a range of zero, which means the measurement is perfectly balanced or aligned, all the way to nine points, which means the measurement is largely imbalanced or misaligned.

Each plane includes three planar measurements. The total score for each plane ranges from zero, meaning there are no misalignments in that plane, to 27, meaning each measurement taken in that plane has a high degree of imbalance of misalignment. So, for three planes, the total score ranges from zero points, which is perfect tri-planar alignment, to 81, which is a body that is severely misaligned.

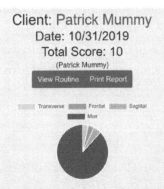

Client: Patrick Mummy
Date: 10/31/2019
Total Score: 10
(Patrick Mummy)

View Routine   Print Report

Transverse   Frontal   Sagittal
Max

(Scale = 0-27 within each plane, 0-81 total possible. Lower is better!)

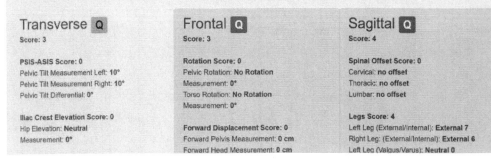

Transverse Q
Score: 3

PSIS-ASIS Score: 0
Pelvic Tilt Measurement Left: **10°**
Pelvic Tilt Measurement Right: **10°**
Pelvic Tilt Differential: **0°**

Iliac Crest Elevation Score: 0
Hip Elevation: **Neutral**
Measurement: **0°**

Frontal Q
Score: 3

Rotation Score: 0
Pelvic Rotation: **No Rotation**
Measurement: **0°**
Torso Rotation: **No Rotation**
Measurement: **0°**

Forward Displacement Score: 0
Forward Pelvis Measurement: **0 cm**
Forward Head Measurement: **0 cm**

Sagittal Q
Score: 4

Spinal Offset Score: 0
Cervical: **no offset**
Thoracic: **no offset**
Lumbar: **no offset**

Legs Score: 4
Left Leg (External/Internal): **External 7**
Right Leg: (External/Internal): **External 6**
Left Leg (Valgus/Varus): **Neutral 0**

From this point, the software automatically creates a suggested sequence of corrective exercises, known as a Routine, which the practitioner can edit, depending on their level of subscription. This sequence is what is then demonstrated to the client to make sure that the client can not only perform the routine correctly, but the results are validated by remeasuring after the session to verify the routine's efficacy. Once the routine has been approved and successful, the delivery of the routine is automatically loaded onto the client's home screen of their mobile device, to a previously downloaded web link that appears as an app, even though it is not a true app. The practitioner can then utilize a series of options that allow for consistent at-home support for the client to make sure they are compliant and successful. Again, there are too many options to demonstrate in this book, but

128

these are the basic features of the AlignSmart Technology™ for the practitioner.

1	*** Static Floor 11 0	
2	Shoulder Rotations (Static Floor) 11 1	
3	Shoulder Rotations (Wall) 12 1	
4	Arm Rotations (Bent Legs) 12 1	
5	Piriformis Stretch (Elevated Crossover) 22 2	
6	TFL Stretch 23 2	
7	Hip Adduction (Extended Floor Position- Elbows) 31 3	
8	Straight Arm Rotations (Kneeling) 61 3	
9	Straight Arm Rotations (Sitting) 72 3	
10	Overhead Extension (Wall Sit) 83 4	
11	Squat (Extended) 83 4	
12	Squat (Full) 83 4	
Add New		+

AlignSmart™ Technology for the Client

As I have mentioned many times in this book, what makes Symmetry successful, besides the patented process, is the consistency of the client performing their routines at home, in between sessions. All the science in the world cannot replace the importance of a client performing their routines at home, and eventually, making it a lifestyle change. The technology that we created is designed specifically to do three things: 1) aid the client in the performing of the exercises with written and video instructions; 2) continual education as the client progresses throughout the phases of treatment; and 3) constant support through our unique messaging system, that not only allows our clients to communicate with us daily while at home, but also to check in with us daily to prove to us that they have performed their routines. I always joke with my clients that I was raised Catholic, so I can guilt the heck out of anyone, but it does work! At each new session, we pull up the client's dashboard and can see how many times they have performed their routines, and if they haven't consistently checked in daily, then we have a talk. And that discussion either ends up as a confession, or that they simply forgot to check in daily, but did perform their routines daily. Either way, it is a great way to ensure the focus of our philosophy, and that again is to teach a person how to fish. Once the client has our icon on their home screen of their mobile device, it is as simple as clicking on it daily to access all these options that are available. We even can send video messages within the app for the clients to get updated information, or to view the latest *Client of the Week* testimonial.

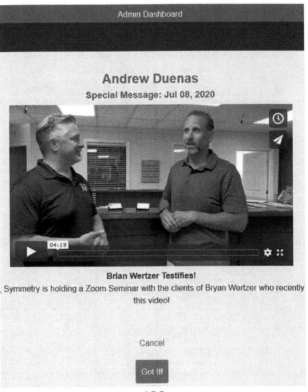

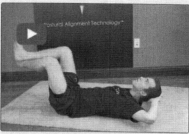

Patrick Mummy
My Routines

Measurement Chart

Score Index

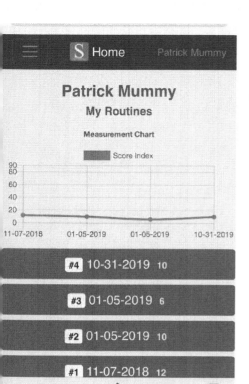

#4	10-31-2019	10
#3	01-05-2019	6
#2	01-05-2019	10
#1	11-07-2018	12

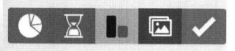

1. Abdominal Crunches (Free)
(2x20)

Special Instructions: **Block@Knees**

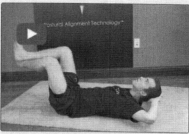

Lying on your back, cross your ankles and lift your legs to a 70-degree position at the hips from the floor keeping your legs slightly bent. With your hands interlaced behind your head, look backwards and lift your elbows, shoulders and head off the floor as one unit using your abdominal muscles, then return to the starting position with your elbows, shoulders and head touching the floor at the same time. Be careful not to

1. Static Floor
(5 Minutes)

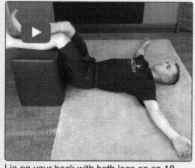

Lie on your back with both legs on an 18-20" block, knees bent to 90 degrees. Keep your arms out to your side with your palms up. Relax your back into the floor and breathe through your diaphragm. Stay in this position for the allotted amount of time.

- Spinal Offset Thoracic

131

Complete Routine   ×

Add Notes: (Optional)

Notes

☐ Notify practitioner

Completed Routine

Cancel

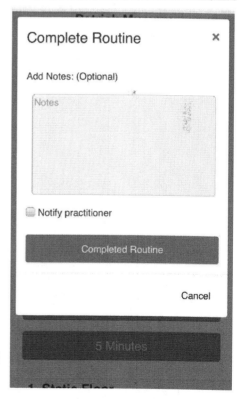

As with the practitioner options, there are too many to discuss all of them in this book, but the general idea is that we hold the client accountable as they go through our program, and technically, for the rest of their lives. Once a client has finished with our program, it is advised that each new month they pick three old routines that they have not performed in a while and rotate daily with the three until the next month. And we send out an automatic email at the beginning of each month for the rest of their lives reminding them to do so. With this general reminder, clients have life-long access to the messaging system as well, so if they run into a bump in the road, or just have a general question, our system is able to support them so that they stay consistent and out of pain!

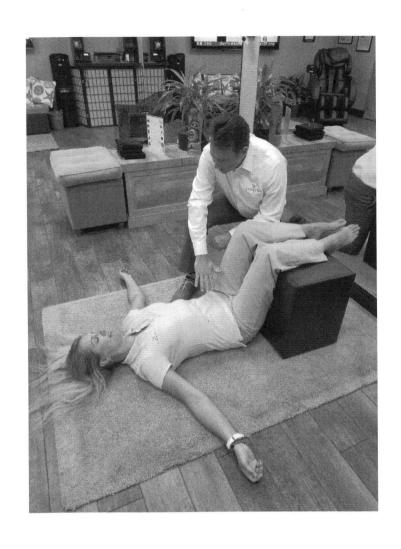

"Every Experience is a Success."

~ Louise Hay, Former Symmetry Client

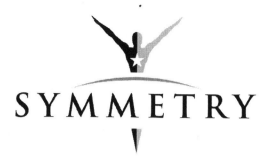

SYMMETRY

TRY IT YOURSELF!

Okay. Hopefully, you have been intrigued thus far to want to delve a little deeper. This is where the self-help portion of the book comes in that I swore I would never do again like my first two books. You see, the problem with self-help books is that they must be generically written to a broad audience and hope that whatever is suggested for you to do will somehow stick and make you feel amazing! It is IMPOSSIBLE for any expert to write a book, sell you on a philosophy, and then give you the magic potion in a book. Even if you have success with these different types of books, and I can give you a list, I guarantee it will be short-lived. Why? Let me explain. There are 12 systems that run the human body. These include:

1. Circulatory system
2. Digestive system
3. Endocrine system
4. Immune system
5. Lymphatic system
6. Nervous system
7. Muscular system
8. Reproductive system
9. Skeletal system
10. Respiratory system

135

11.   Urinary system

12.   Integumentary system

The human body contains of over 100 trillion cells. The human brain contains about 100 billion nerve cells. In the skeletal and muscular system alone, there are 856 parts that run these systems, and thousands of parts for the remaining systems. There are so many variables to the human body that it is impossible to understand you, the reader, to the extent that I would confidently know how to treat you with this book! So, am I an expert in my field? I suppose some would argue this, but I am not about to tell you that if you perform the following example routines, you will be cured of your ailments. Yes, to check off my legal box, consult with your doctor first. However, I will tell you that in my 25 years in this field, I can confidently give you a couple of choices of corrective sequences that fall within the general margins of what most people present to me when they first come into our clinic. Let me paint a clearer picture. The average client comes in for a full year in our program, assessed sixteen times during this period, and is given a unique sequence each time based upon the system I have. It takes at least three months for the body to start showing consistent holding patterns, and then three months of strengthening to make sure it holds. Then, we educate our clients on how to maintain this momentum and structure.

Why do I say this? Because it is only one percent of one percent of the population that is motivated enough to even take a system presented in a book, actually complete the entire process presented in such a book, and then implement it consistently for the rest of their life. So, experience the following routines with the understanding that this is just a taste of how to get your body to start releasing your years of compensation patterns. What you will more than likely feel with the first routine is a positive result right away. This is mainly due to unwinding the Transverse Plane issues that most people show, so the tension caused by this pattern will usually give you immediate relief.

Do this routine for at least one to two weeks, twice a day if you are motivated, and then switch to the second one.

The second routine you will not feel as great as you did with the first. This is because most of your large disparities will be corrected in the first routine, which gives you the most unwinding, resulting in the most relief. But it will be temporary as your body then adjusts as the new layers of dysfunction rear their ugly head. Our recommendation after this is to either find an AlignSmart™ specialist near you to complete the entire process or take the two routines and rotate between them on a semi-weekly basis. This will at least keep you in somewhat control over your issues and allow for you to have some consistent correction to rely on every other day. But it will not take you to the Promised Land. Nothing ever great in life is easy to achieve. You have just been conditioned to rely on the experts so that you cannot ever really get better, and so that you keep contributing your hard-earned dollars to the pit of recycled wellness. It is capitalism at its best!

If you run into an exercise or two that are either contradicted by your doctor's advice, or you just don't feel good while doing it, either skip the exercise or give an AlignSmart™ specialist a call to help you out. We have 400+ corrective exercises to choose from if you were to go through the entire program, so we can certainly help you out with suggesting an alternative exercise. However, please make sure that you are performing the routines in the sequence they were given. It does make a difference.

ROUTINE #1

Static Floor: Lie on your back with both legs on a chair that is 18-20 inches high, knees bent to 90-degrees. Keep your arms out to your side with your palms up. Relax your back into the floor and breathe through your diaphragm. Stay in this position for five minutes.

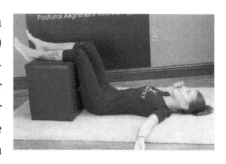

Hip Rotations (Static Floor): Lying on your back with your knees and hips bent at 90-degrees and feet on an 18-inch block or chair, place your feet together with your toes pulled back, heels halfway on the block. Keeping your feet straight and

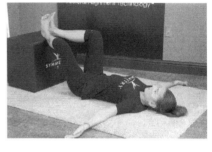

together slowly spread your knees apart while pivoting on the inside of your feet as they stay together. Do not let your feet separate as your knees widen apart and try to keep them flexed throughout the motion. Your practitioner may have you place a six-inch block in between your feet for more support. Perform two sets of 10 to 20 repetitions.

TFL Stretch (Bent Leg): Start on your back with your legs straight out, knees and feet hip-width and pointing up to the ceiling. Keep your arms straight out from your side, with your palms up. Tighten one leg and flex your foot back, raise the

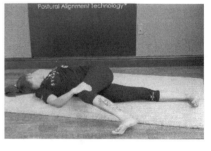

other leg to 90-degrees at the hip and then bend that knee to 90-degrees. Take your opposite hand and reach to the outside of the elevated knee and pull your entire leg across your body without the opposite shoulder rising off the floor. Make sure that your other leg stays tight, feet flexed at the ankle. Look to the opposite direction and keep your stomach and upper torso relaxed. Breathe! Hold for 30 seconds to 1 minute per side and then switch.

Shoulder Rotations (Kneeling):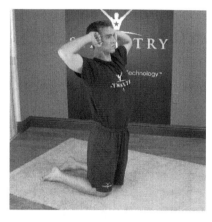
Kneeling, induce an arch in your lower back by rolling your hips forward and not by leaning your torso back. Position your hands with your knuckles on your temples, palms facing to the front. Keeping your knuckles on your temples and your wrists from bending, bring your elbows together and touch in front of your chest, but chin-high, with your palms now facing each other. Try to keep your head still by not bobbing it back and forth as you try and touch your elbows together. Then separate your elbows by pulling your arms back, squeezing your shoulder blades together and then repeat. Keep your stomach relaxed by inhaling as you separate your elbows and exhaling as you bring your elbows together. Perform two sets of 10 to 20 repetitions.

Extended Ankle Abduction: Start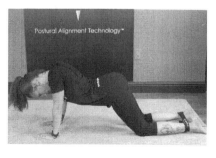
with your hands and knees hip-width and perpendicular to floor. Walk your hands forward four to six inches and allow your shoulders to reposition over your hands without moving your knees on the floor. With your hips now in front of your knees, allow your back to sway, shoulder blades to collapse together, and head to drop, but keep your

elbows locked. While holding this position, press out on a strap hip-width at your ankles for one second and then release. Feel the contraction on the outside of your hips. Breathe and relax your stomach. In between each set, keep your hands in the same position and push your body back to stretch out your lower back. Perform two sets of 10 to 20 repetitions.

Hip Adduction (Sitting): Sitting with your knees bent to 90 degrees, place a six-inch block between your knees. With your feet straight, arms to your side, press in against the block and release for one second, relaxing your stomach and shoulders. Exhale as you press in and inhale as you relax. Allow your back to be slightly arched by rolling your pelvis forward and your 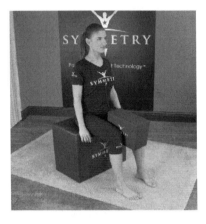 shoulders pulled together without shrugging. Perform two sets of 10 to 20 repetitions.

ROUTINE #2

Static Floor: Lie on your back with both legs on a chair that is18-20 inches high, knees bent to 90-degrees. Keep your arms out to your side with your palms up. Relax your back into the floor and breathe through your diaphragm. Stay in this position for five minutes.

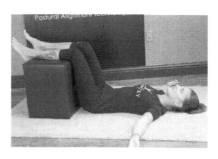

Hip Rotations (Wall): Lying on your back with your knees and hips bent at 90-degrees, place your feet hip-width and straight on a wall. Keeping your feet straight (Almost pigeon-toed) slowly spread your knees apart while pivoting on the

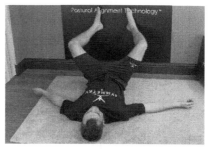

outside of your feet keeping your heels on the wall, then bring your knees together and then repeat. After each set, reposition your feet correctly on the wall if necessary. Keep your stomach relaxed and rest in between each set for a duration of two deep breaths. Perform two sets of 10 to 20 repetitions.

Piriformis Stretch (Crossover): Lie on your back with your knees bent, feet on the floor, and hip-width. Cross your right ankle to left knee and pivot off the outside of your left foot and rotate your right foot and left knee to the floor as one

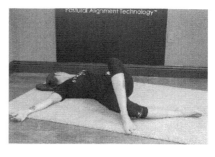

unit. Make sure to not let your left foot slide in as you rotate on its side. Keeping your right foot flat on floor, press your right knee slightly away feeling a stretch on the outside of the right hip. Place arms out to side, relax your shoulders and stomach and look the opposite direction. Hold for 30 seconds to one minute per side.

Arm Glides (Inverted Wall): Lie on your back with legs straight up on a wall, feet hip-width apart. With your quads tight, position your body away from wall, if necessary, so that your tailbone and back rests on the floor. Keeping your knees pointed straight off the wall and toes flexed back, feel a stretch in 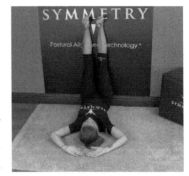 hamstrings and calves. Keep your feet flat as if you were trying to hold a drink on them. Relax your stomach and hold this position. Proceed to bend your elbows at 90-degrees placing your arms and back of hands on the floor. Maintaining a 90-degree angle, slowly raise your arms overhead until your hands touch. Keep your elbows, forearms, and hands slightly pressed into floor. Return to starting position and repeat for allotted number of repetitions. Be sure to inhale and allow your back to arch as you reach arms overhead. As this first position becomes easier, glide arms higher by touching hands further above your head. Relax in between each set and rest for the duration of two deep breaths. Perform two sets of 10 repetitions.

Hip Rotations (Extended Floor Position): Start with your hands and knees hip-width and perpendicular to the floor. Walk your hands forward four to six inches and allow your shoulders to reposition over your hands without moving knees on 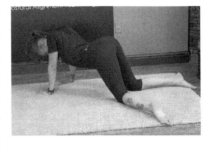 floor. Let your back sway with shoulder blades together and arms straight. Proceed to slide your feet apart while staying in contact with the floor, pivoting off your knees, feeling the rotation from your hip joint. Separate your feet as much as you can, feeling the stretch in your hips, then bring your feet back together and repeat, keeping your form throughout the exercise. In between sets, push your buttocks back to your heels to stretch out your back for a few seconds, then repeat. Perform two sets of 10 to 20 repetitions.

Hip Abduction (Static): Sitting tall by rolling your pelvis forward with your knees bent to 90-degrees, place a strap around your knees either together or hip-width. With your feet straight, arms to your side, press out against the strap and hold for one to two minutes, relaxing your stomach and shoulders. Breathe.

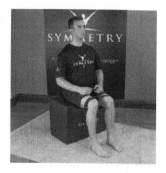

Wall Sit: With your low back against a wall, slowly walk your feet away from the wall. Keeping your feet hip-width apart and straight ahead, slide down the wall until your knees are at 90-degree angles or just above. Press your low back into the wall by placing the weight on your heels and not your toes. Keep your stomach and shoulders relaxed. Feel in your thighs and quads.

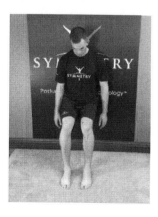

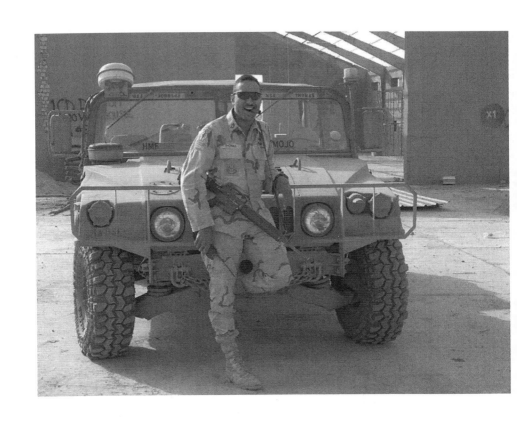

*"Like a fine wine gets better with time,
so does Symmetry with your body."*

~ Anthony Joseph Thomas

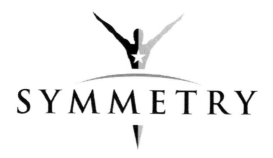

SYMMETRY

SUCCESS!

I have been blessed and fortunate enough to travel this path to become pain-free. It has indeed been the road less traveled. I would have never experienced what I did if I had gone the traditional route. Most of my college friends went on to get their masters or PhDs in some healthcare field, such as chiropractic or physical therapy, and are doing fine in life. This route has been riskier, but with great risk comes great reward. Every day I get to interact with people who have been sullied by the healthcare system and left with dismal choices. When I see my clients progressing to long-term wellness, it is the greatest joy to hear them explain how it feels to be out of pain, and that they realize that they did it themselves. I get thanked every day, but the reality, and what I tell them, is that they did all the hard work. We just bossed them around, with lots of love, education and motivation, of course.

Our mission now is to certify every willing practitioner out there who believes that we as practitioners are just the conduit to showing people how to become well again. What I love about the AlignSmart™ system is that it provides the tools and education for people who are tired of being sick and tired by giving them the real opportunity to become healthy again and set and reach goals they once thought were impossible. I live this every day myself. My love now is playing basketball. Every time I play, I spend most of the time doing my routine before I play, because I know what I know. I have been playing at my gym now for 10 years, and knock on wood, I have avoided serious injury because I prepare myself daily and have no fear anymore of pushing my body to its limits. Most everyone else shows up, grabs a ball, and starts shooting. And if they do stretch, it is the same thing each time. They just do not know what they do not know. I want to educate the world as to why this system should be the main source of wellness, in all models. If you do not know what to do and why to do it daily, then at the end of the day, you too are just guessing as to how to become well again.

Being in this business for as long as I have, you end up finding people who have the same values and the same mission. One of our latest opportunities we have been fortunate enough to affiliate ourselves with is the Parkinson's community. My great friend Kevin Quinn owns a few franchises called *Rock Steady Boxing*; a program designed specifically for those afflicted with Parkinson's disease. Kevin called me up one day and told me he was referring one of his newest members, Ralph, who came to him one day to join his gym, but as Kevin recalled, "I had no idea what I was going to do with Ralph, because he couldn't even stand up by himself without assistance". I remember Kevin asking me if he thought I could help him. I have never said no to anyone because of my faith in people, not just our patented system. So, Ralph came in, and Kevin was right, Ralph was severely affected by this disease. Not only was he unable to stand or move by himself, his speech was noticeably diminished, which is one of the symptoms of Parkinson's. The first thing we do with new clients is take their pictures. What you see here is Ralph's posterior view, but what you do not see is his assistant Connie who was standing just outside of the frame. Once we placed Ralph into position, I told Connie to let him go, we took the picture, and then she immediately grabbed him so he would not fall over.

One of the biggest lessons I have learned being in this business is that your bad situation is always trumped by someone else's bad situation. However, certain people handle bad situations with amazing

146

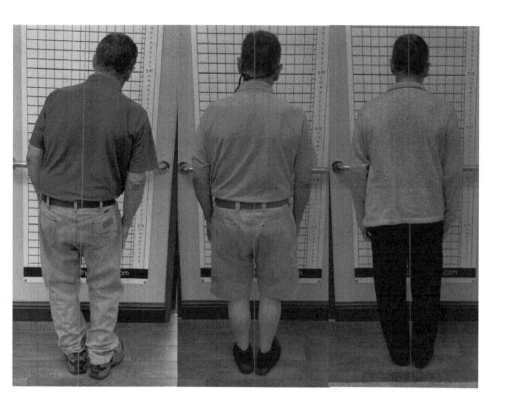

resolve, and the Parkinson's community is no exception. Every Parkinson's client I have worked with is the happiest, most polite, respectful, and motivated client I have ever worked with. When Ralph first came to our office, I knew right away that he was going to be a success with our program because his entire demeanor was that of a champion. After his first measurement Ralph scored a 60 out of 81 possible points, which is extremely high on the scale. What you see in his pictures is the progression from his first session, to his sixth (six weeks), to his 12th session, (eight months). From his first session to his sixth, I asked Kevin to excuse Ralph from *Rock Steady* classes for me to get Ralph firmly engrained in the Symmetry process. I do not ask this of all my Parkinson's clients, but in Ralph's case I did not have a choice. Kevin understood what I was trying to do and so he placated me.

When Ralph returned to Kevin's gym six-weeks after he started our program, I received a phone call from a man who sounded like he had witnessed a miracle. We interviewed Kevin, which is on our Facebook page, where you will hear him explain the difference he saw in Ralph when he first came back. Not only was Ralph able to move on his own, but the way he moved was nothing short of a miracle. Moving, punching, with force. Ralph's speech improved, so much so, you no longer must move in close to try and understand him. His entire outlook is incredible and just wonderful to witness. The reason I created Symmetry was to place the power and control back in the hands of those who thought it could never happen again.

Testimonials

The following testimonials are from some of my favorite clients. They indeed are the reason we do what we do. Enjoy!

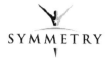

SYMMETRY

"I am a 42-year-old veteran of the United States Army. I spent 22 years in active duty. During that time, I worked as a paratrooper-mechanic, infantryman, and drill instructor. The activities I participated in daily included but were not limited to 4 to 10 mile runs in the morning with calisthenics. Four, eight, and 12-mile foot marches with 60-pound rucksack, heavy lifting in every conceivable position on a daily basis, airborne operations with combat equipment exceeding 265 pounds and the ever faithful standard of putting your weapon into operation once you land, recover your equipment and double-time it to the assembly area with all that equipment on your person. Hopefully, one could find it in the darkness in a reasonable amount of time. What is the bottom line? You had to be mentally and physically tough to endure these rigors.

After 22 years of training troops and doing Uncle Sam's business abroad, I retired a back-broken individual who woke daily to sharp pains which ran up my back and down the back of my legs. In x-rays, my L-4 and 5 were black! I thought I would need surgery and spend the rest of my life taking medication. Little did I know that my life would take a drastic change for the better in December of 2006. The first time I was told about Symmetry by Patrick Mummy, I was skeptical. If there were such a solution for my back pain, the military would be an intricate and developmental part of it. After all, I served honorably and deserve the best! After getting measured and going through my first routine, I will admit I felt better. However, I was still very skeptical that exercises would alleviate my pain. I was given a Symmetry routine and continued to follow that routine's guidelines until I finished. Then I went on to my second routine and then third. I have not felt this limber and agile since I was a young paratrooper in the 82nd Airborne Division. It is amazing!

I can tell you quite honestly that I quit doing the routine once. But that lasted all of 10 days, until my back pain became so unbearable that I had to restart my routine. Two days after restarting, the pain was totally gone. Why do I sing the unsolicited praises of something I have to pay for? Because it works and I think everyone who experiences back pain should learn of this program and do it to improve their standard of living. Back pain can be stressful. Today, I am stress free. Thank you, Patrick, and Symmetry!"

~Joseph A. Thomas, Master Sergeant, United States Army (Retired)

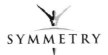

SYMMETRY

"When it comes to raffle prizes or drawings, I never win. I just do not. In the spring of 2014, my luck changed at a charity golf tournament. I threw some tickets into a basket for this item called "Symmetry, Postural Alignment Technology™" because it looked interesting. The next thing I knew, they were calling my number. I won! At the time, I did not care that it was for Symmetry, I was simply happy to *finally* win something!

After the thrill of victory passed, my Symmetry package sat in an envelope on my desk at home for a few months. One day while cleaning, I found it and decided to call and make an appointment. I am always a little skeptical about new approaches to health and wellness. And, as a busy wife, mother and business owner, finding time to do something like this is always problematic. But this package was worth over $1,000, so I thought I might as well check it out. One phone call and a week later, I walked into the place that would turn my current perspective of my structural wellbeing upside down.

The first thing I discovered is Symmetry is a happy place; like the kind of happy you find among good friends. Seriously. Upon entering a pleasantly decorated office with big windows, I was greeted by the larger-than-life enthusiasm of Symmetry founder, Patrick Mummy. After approaching me like he had known me for years and offering me tea, we proceeded to chat. He asked me a series of questions about my health concerns, exercise habits and physical pain level. He explained the theory behind Symmetry and how having our bodies in alignment eliminates a lot of physical health problems and chronic pain issues. Patrick then pulled out this funky little measuring device he developed called a Postural Alignment Tool, which measures specific misalignments. Still skeptical, I listened. He went on to tell me about how this device works and how I would be able to correct my misalignment with exercise routines I would do at home. It made sense and sounded easy enough, but did it work, and did I need it?

Then it began...the measuring, the evaluation, and the truth about my personal symmetry situation. Patrick measured my alignment and entered my numbers into Symmetry's patented software program. This software calculates your measurements three-dimensionally to determine postural issues and the specific exercises needed to correct each one. As they were taking measurements of my spine, hips and shoulders, and evaluating the placement of my knees, feet and head, I kept thinking, "How bad can I be? I can't be that out of line, can I?" After it was all over, I was about to enter the first phase of the Symmetry school of humility. What is worse, they had the photos to prove it. In addition to the numbers revealed by the software, they also take a few photos of you in front of a grid so they can visually point out to you where you are misaligned. It is important to note they do all this evaluating with you fully dressed; perfect for modest gals like me.

It is a good thing I was sitting down when the software kicked out alignment numbers and they showed me the photos. I was a misaligned, lopsided, forward-tilting, knock-kneed mess. On a scale of 0 to 27 with 0 being perfect alignment, I scored a 24 in the Transverse category (elevation of hips, shoulders); an 11 in the Frontal category (body rotation); and 15 in the Sagittal category (offset of spine, head, shoulders, knees, feet) for a total score of 50. Yikes! What's worse, Patrick knew exactly what I was experiencing from a pain and physical symptoms standpoint without me having to tell him. I was like an open book – I had been officially busted.

After swallowing my pride and conceding the fact that I had some serious alignment problems, he proceeded to devise my first exercise routine. The Symmetry exercise routine is based on two things: 1) where you need correction and 2) how much time you have each day to commit to the routine. Based on my input, Patrick created a 15-minute routine that I was to complete twice daily. To make sure you do everything correctly, you receive the exercises on an amazing app, do the routine under a watchful eye at the office, and if you still have questions, you can watch video demonstrations on the app. Patrick's background is in athletic training, so the exercises reflect his knowledge of the human musculoskeletal system and are directly connected to a multitude of symptoms exposed in the evaluation.

Enter the second phase of the Symmetry school of humility. Exercises that looked easy on paper quickly brought me to my knees (literally) when I had to lie on the floor and contort myself into all sorts of ridiculous positions. This was only made more challenging by repetitive motions that worked various parts of my body into exhaustion; "feel the burn" type of exhaustion. I have been physically fit my entire life, so why was this so hard and awkward? All the while, Patrick smiled with one of those "We told you so!" type grins that made me want to prove to them that I really could do this. As I got in my car to drive home, I decided I would give it a few weeks and see for myself if this was the real deal.

Two weeks later, I returned for my first evaluation. I quickly got the tangible proof I needed in my sore body and my next set of numbers.

My total score plummeted from a 50 to a 30. The process of breaking years of alignment issues from sitting at work, playing sports, carrying toddlers on my hip, lifting heavy objects, and who knows what else, was happening. My body was willing to correct itself, but I had to be willing to make the commitment to continue. For the next two months, I went to Symmetry every two weeks for a check-up. Each time I went back, I would get measured, we would discuss symptoms, and I would come home with a new set of exercises. Unfortunately, the exercises did not get easier nor did finding the time to do them. But discipline is the main reason Symmetry works. If you do not do the work, you cannot make the corrections.

As I write this, after I began what I like to call the raffle-winning Symmetry experiment, I am now in the maintenance phase. My numbers are now 3 (Transverse), 5 (Frontal) and 3 (Sagittal) for a total score of 11, which if you do not know what this means- it is great! What am I feeling? I am feeling a lot less pain (I have Fibromyalgia), my hips don't make a "popping" noise anymore, my knees aren't so turned in, my spine is straight, and when I run, my body feels 10 years younger. Do I still feel some soreness with my exercises? Yes. My body is still correcting itself and I am okay with that. I feel a sense of accomplishment knowing that I am taking charge of my physical health with non-invasive technology that is helping me now AND preventing issues down the road. Feeling good today is nice, but knowing I can prevent future hip surgery, pain medication, and back issues is even better. Even though Symmetry's exercises are hard and make me look ridiculous, I will take it!

Having my body in alignment has improved my speed and recovery for distance running. Any runner will tell you that as you pile on the miles training for a race, you run the risk of some type of injury. I have become so much stronger due to Symmetry that I decided to increase the intensity of my training to qualify for the Boston Marathon. What I once thought was impossible became a reality! On December 4, 2016, I ran a Boston Qualifying (BQ) time of 3:36:13. It does not end there. In February of 2017, I ran my first ultra-marathon on a trail, a 50k distance (31 miles), and finished 47th out of more than 250 runners. And I could walk the next day! Simply put, Symmetry is the platform that enables your body to achieve its potential. You must have alignment coincide with training and diet to be at your best.

Do I now understand why Symmetry is such a happy place and why Patrick and his associates are so excited about their jobs? Absolutely. What Patrick has created in Symmetry is a pathway to better structural and physical health for the long-term. He challenges the traditional paradigm of the quick fix, over-medicating, and fad solutions. Symmetry is not about being temporary; it is about lasting change and empowerment to feel and look better. If you are seeking a real difference in your wellness, do not hesitate to put your tickets in the Symmetry basket. You might just discover you won the lottery."

~Melissa Copley

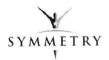

SYMMETRY

"As a recipient of the Symmetry AlignSmart™ system, I have been able to make adjustments to my body and sustain my level of activity in the gym 4 to 5 times a week as well as increase my performance on the Golf course. Most importantly, I have been able to increase the quality of my life by being able to put my body in the optimal position in gravity, thus allowing gravity to be my friend and not foe.

As a 27-year Holistic Health practitioner, certified structural integrative therapist, and injury treatment specialist, I have seen the efficacy of my treatments and client base increase upwards of 50%. Adding Symmetry AlignSmart™ programming and measurements to show exactly what posture, strength, and stretching components are needed along with comparative analysis and pre/post evaluations all has proven invaluable methods to use. Without question, Symmetry should be a modality in every form of Physical Therapy."

~Kelley Schlager, HHP, Certified structural integrationist/Rolfer, CHEK practitioner, Certified Symmetry Professional Practitioner

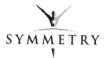

SYMMETRY

"Throughout my professional running career, I won multiple national titles and was ranked amongst the finest runners in the world. Once I retired, I knew I needed to tend to my body so I could have a good quality of life, post-athletics. Symmetry has been a big part of the wellness recipe I follow. Now, at the age of 41, I feel better than ever. And when I have women half my age ask me how I stay in such great shape; I know I'm doing something right!"

~Milena Glusac, 7-time NCAA All American; 3-time US National Champion; and Top 10 finishes at Boston and New York Marathons

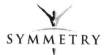

SYMMETRY

"I was in my mid-forties, swimming with the master's team and doing hot yoga when old injuries came back to haunt me. My right shoulder was grinding during swim workouts and increasing pain in my right hip was resulting in a limp. How could I maintain a healthy active lifestyle if I could not walk and could not swim without pain? A medical doctor who had been helped by Patrick referred me to Symmetry. Today I am pain-free and have flexibility, which is a good thing because I must keep up with my 7 kids. Since the chronic pain is behind me, I have been able to move more and have lost weight. I love being in control of my treatment by doing my routine regularly. I am no longer tied to the chiropractor's office. Everyone that I have referred to Symmetry has experienced sweet relief, including my very skeptical, inactive, MD husband. It works!"

~Lesley Lidge

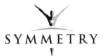
SYMMETRY

"I discovered Symmetry in the spring of 2015 in a time of pure desperation. I had chronic patellar pain in both knees, on and off sciatica in my left hip, pain in my right upper back, and tendonitis in both forearms. During this time, I was a personal trainer at a sports club and a strength coach for a boys' gymnastics team, and although I had a reputation for being obsessed with rehabilitation and posture, it was my own body that was constantly falling apart! In addition to this, I had a bachelor's degree in Exercise Science and was looking to start Physical Therapy school in the fall. But for all my investment in continued education, internships, research, and work experience, I could not get my own body out of pain. The system from which I was learning, was missing something critical.

I was so desperate for relief that I even started writing my own book, a compilation of my experiences and knowledge regarding rehabilitation of chronic injuries. Not surprisingly, the realization that I came to during this process was that postural dysfunction causes muscular compensation patterns to form throughout the body, which in turn causes inefficient movement, thus damage to the joints.

Around this time, I was introduced to Patrick by one of the gymnastics coaches I worked with. My first thought was: "It's too simple! These exercises are too easy to make lasting postural changes..." But after some time of doing my Symmetry routine and examining the logic behind the measurement and sequencing process, I had to admit Patrick was about 20 years ahead of me on the same journey I was so strongly set upon. And he understood my struggle from the very start! The fact that he experienced the same shortcomings of our healthcare system and created Symmetry out of necessity to heal his own injuries remains one of my greatest inspirations.

Fast forward to Fall of 2016, I am not the same person I used to be! I have been out of chronic pain for over a year. Since starting work with Symmetry, I have seen hundreds of individuals who, just like myself, were out of options and looking for a last-ditch effort to get their lives back on track. Symmetry for me represents so much more than just posture and pain relief. It is a symbol of not giving up. It is a symbol of the relentless pursuit of the scientific method, the determination to not settle for mediocre or incomplete results that are just good enough, but to go above and beyond to find out the innermost causes of a problem so it can be addressed effectively. Thank you, Patrick Mummy, for never giving up."

~Andrew "AJ" Juntunen, B.S. Exercise Science, CSCS, SPP

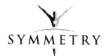

SYMMETRY

"I was a ballet dancer and in pain since the age of 12 and diagnosed with Scoliosis. Nothing I tried helped my pain, so I just learned to live with it. I became a Certified Massage Therapist wanting to help others when I could not help myself, and after 10 years, I was physically exhausted and in more pain after giving multiple massages every day. I found Symmetry in 2014 and this process has changed my life! Symmetry made such an impact on me that I have changed careers and am now a certified AlignSmart™ therapist and the Director of Sales at Symmetry. I wish I would have known about Symmetry when I was a massage therapist because I would have referred all my clients to Symmetry to help them rid themselves of pain permanently. I am no longer in pain nor have Scoliosis and I also lost a significant amount of weight. My outlook and quality of life has completely changed, and I love living pain free!"

~Lee Anne Carson, CMT, Certified Symmetry Professional Practitioner

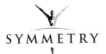

SYMMETRY

"My name is Andy Rocklin and I discovered Symmetry for Health back in 2011. Throughout my life, I have always been an active person who played many sports, including competitive soccer. In 1997 and 1998 I had two knee surgeries that replaced my meniscus and fixed my MCL and ACL. Since those two surgeries, I had recurring issues in one of my knees, thus causing one to be weaker than the other. My knee would hurt. I would pull muscles and experience chronic lower back tightness. My doctor, who was doing her best to help me with my ongoing issues, recommended that I see Patrick Mummy, as he specializes in fixing ailments like my own.

So, I visited the Symmetry office and on my first evaluation I scored a 68, which is not particularly good at all! He explained how his system works and why I was constantly hurting in one area or the other. Being a highly motivated person, I like the fact that the treatment was in my own hands and that I can do the exercises on my own time, as often as I could and therefore help myself get better. I think it is one of the best parts about the system, that the patient helps themselves. Symmetry routines can be done anywhere and anytime. So, I went through the program and started feeling much better. I was and still am injury free for over 9 years now.

However, I was incredibly surprised to hear that Symmetry was not a house-hold name, and that he had not trained thousands of practitioners in this technology. So, I offered Patrick my help and knowledge to take this out into the world so that hundreds of thousands of people could get help and benefit from this amazing system. That is when the partnership was born and grew from there. Fast forward seven years and we are finally introducing our new technology to the world. Our goal is to train Symmetry Practitioners all over the world to help as many people as possible enjoy a pain-free, healthy lifestyle.

I cannot say enough about Patrick and the amazing technology he created. I have seen many people walk away from pain, cancel their surgeries and enjoy an overall better quality of life."

~Andy Rocklin, Entrepreneur

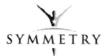

SYMMETRY

"I am grateful I gave Symmetry a try. I have a highly active life and love my various workouts. I started walking with a hitch, as I put it, and began getting bad hip pain. After trying standard pain relief options, I reluctantly got a cortisone shot. That only took away the shooting pain, but the hip pain and hitch were still there and very painful!

I went in to visit Patrick and he suggested that I stop my workouts for a few weeks and let his Symmetry process start working. Not wanting to really stop my progress for my race training, I was very skeptical, but I decided this was the time to get better, and to listen to my body yelling at me so I stopped my workouts for a couple of weeks. About one and a half months into faithfully doing the individualized routines that Patrick set up for me, I had my Spartan Sprint Race. During the race, I was completing an obstacle that normally had my hip in an upset. I was feeling like something was missing and realized it was the intense pain! The pain level had greatly diminished. Fast forward 4-months and five races later, my hip had no pain. My running time went down since my legs and hips could move the proper way, with no hitch in my step. Another bonus was my pinky and index fingers no longer fall asleep. In the past I went to my doctor and they wanted to do surgery to alleviate the fingers falling asleep and tingling sensations. After going through Symmetry, I am happy to say I have not had any sleeping fingers or tingling. Walking into Symmetry is always a wonderful experience for me. I love all the staff and they have all been extremely helpful. I highly suggest that you see them and see how they can help you too!"

~Crystal

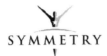

SYMMETRY

"My name is Andrew Bloch. Amongst other things, I am a Physical Therapist as well as a licensed Acupuncturist. I met Patrick 6 years ago at a symposium in San Diego. I remember distinctly walking by his booth and seeing his system of corrective exercises up on his 44" flat screen. I gravitated immediately to Patrick's product because I just listened to a conference on qualitative postural analysis which left me wanting something different to help me identify potential postural dysfunction. As Patrick began to explain to me how he had created an entire patented system of corrective exercises through measuring posture and creating a quantifiable report to not only explain his treatment protocols, but verify and validate them from session to session, I was very impressed. This type of advanced technology is sorely missing in the Physical Technology world. Four months later my business partner, Dr. Brian Paris, and I flew Patrick out to take our clinic through his certification program.

For 9 years now, we have utilized the AlignSmart™ system in our office. Not only does it validate our evaluations for insurance, but more importantly validates the treatments I use for my patients. Using Reflexive Pattern Technology™, a system that I created for immediate pain relief, I then have an incredible postural measurement report each session along with the corrective exercise portion of the AlignSmart system, which allows the added benefit of my treatments to hold for a much longer period of time. Also, the emphasis is now transferred to my patients to become proactive in their own treatment by knowing exactly what to do on their own in between their visits with me!

As a healthcare practitioner, both traditional and non-traditional, it is imperative that practitioner's move from qualitative to quantitative data and then use this data to allow a client to be involved in the process of getting well. Symmetry's AlignSmart™ technology is the wave of the future, so catch it now and don't be left behind."

~Andrew Bloch, MSPT, L.Ac; President, Advanced Spine & Wellness Center Creator of Reflexive Pattern Technology™

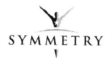

SYMMETRY

"I've known Patrick for over 20 years when a colleague recommended, I see him for back pain. My surgeon friend had a slipped disc that was referred for surgery. After participating in Symmetry not only was my friend back in the operating room but he was skiing within six months! Although my back pain was not as bad, I had pain with everyday activities like driving, bending over to examine patients and sitting at my computer. After three sessions with Patrick, my pain was gone. I was able to participate in my first sprint triathlon. Within 4-months, I was pain free! Patrick's postural alignment therapies, assessments, and exercise program make sense and work well. I've trusted Symmetry to help many family, friends and colleagues that I have referred over the years."

~Linda Smith, M.D., FAAP

"Patrick Mummy relieved my pain when I first came to him. In addition, I also saw a huge increase in my strength, so I could tolerate the exercises I wanted in my life, such as walks and ballroom dancing. Out of my holistic medical practice, I refer a lot of patients for Symmetry work who have had VERY quick relief of their pain. I think the work that Patrick Mummy does has accurate biomechanics and physics as its basis, and out of that can really give people an individualized program that supports their strengthening over time. It also is extremely complementary to any individual body work they might have like chiropractic, massage or cranial sacral which can be temporary, momentary treatments. The person has control of **his/her** own improvements daily to correct their structure, maintain strength and achieve their personal physical goals!"

~Kelly Sutton, MD, Raphael Medicine + Therapies, PC

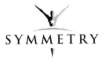

SYMMETRY

"In over 30 years as a Chiropractic Wellness Provider, I have been exposed to many different forms of spinal exercise and gimmicks relative to spinal recovery and rehabilitation. Some of those methods are useful and effective, and I routinely use elements of these approaches as an aspect of our spinal corrective protocols. In 2014, I was introduced to a new systematic approach to postural correction called Symmetry for Health. I was intrigued as one of my stubborn, chronic pain clients had recently received great results from this approach. As is customary for me, I decided to check it out for myself from a patient's perspective. As a new client, I was impressed by the technology behind their assessment and was even more impressed by the results I achieved with the unique, specific rehab protocols they suggested for me. I love that it is mostly self-guided and feel their web-based platform is revolutionary for the rehab and postural correction industry.

I routinely refer my clients to Symmetry for Health to effectively balance and strengthen their body so ultimately, they hold the corrective adjustments we perform on them. If you are not holding your adjustments and are looking for an approach that is corrective and effective, check out Symmetry for Health."

~Dr. Ron Simms, D.C., CEO of Back to Health Chiropractic

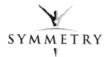

SYMMETRY

"I found Symmetry when I was at an all-time low. We were a year into the Great Recession and my back went out. This would be manageable except that doing massages and running my small three-room massage clinic now looked like an impossibility. Somehow, amid my tears, fears and anger, my dear friend Angie managed to calm me down. She put me on the floor and took me through two Symmetry™ exercises that *immediately* took my back pain away.

I was stunned. That night I kept looking for and expecting the pain to return... but it just did not. I knew I had to know more about Symmetry™ so I looked online and began a journey that night that I will be forever thankful I started. Once I looked deeper, I decided I needed to schedule an appointment with Patrick to go through the full Symmetry™ experience. I will never forget him laughing at my pain and telling me he did not care – and he was right! I had been trained for my entire career to chase the pain but never to get to the root of it and correct the cause.

The AlignSmart™ system does this and so much more. I have never found a more complete system of health care than what Patrick has created. Not only did I receive compassionate and educated care, I learned how to take care of my own body in a totally new and empowering way. Symmetry has taught me that I do not need to suffer. That growing older does not mean accepting aches and pains as a way of life. It has taught me that I can literally control how I feel on any given day. For this and more, I am eternally grateful.

Once I stopped being a Symmetry patient, I knew I needed to become a practitioner.

I've personally witnessed amazing transformations in people that have literally changed their lives - from massage therapists finally having that Aha moment to Physical Therapists and Acupuncturists getting excited again about caring for their patients. Seeing their renewed joy at being able to provide health *care* again only fueled my passion for this work. As a practitioner, I have seen people break down in tears in front of me from sheer relief. Ten years of pain vanishing in a few minutes is truly the norm with this work.

Patrick's generous and loving nature is infused in this work- his demeanor cannot be separated from the work he does. I believe that this is what takes Symmetry above simply being another health care modality to be a complete health care system. I can give no higher recommendation. Do this and you will experience love for your body, work, and sharing Symmetry with others. Being able to help the people we love is a universal desire at the root of our nature. With Symmetry, you'll be able to do that and more."

~Angel Martinez, CMT, SPP

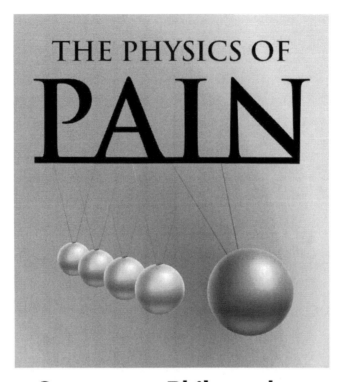

Symmetry Philosophy, Module 1

"The secret of getting ahead is getting started."

~ Mark Twain

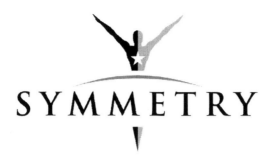

TRAINING AND CERTIFICATION

Symmetry for Health has offered certification courses for practitioners since 2001. In 2015, these courses were put on hold to develop a full online academic curriculum so that anyone, anywhere, can be certified and now licensed as a Symmetry Practitioner. In 2020, we launched our updated curriculum!

Following are the details of the courses that are now online (eCourses) and available to anyone, anywhere, to become certified and licensed in this system I have developed over the past 25 years. If you are a licensed practitioner already, then you may be eligible to bypass our first two modules and directly use our AlignSmart™ app to access our database of corrective exercises. If you are looking for a different career in healthcare, or to enhance your current practice, then these courses are where you would need to start. Please go to https://symmetryalignsmart.com/certification for more information.

Symmetry Philosophy- This is our introductory course and covers the material in this book as well as interactive videos and discussions.

Symmetry Technician I (Intern) - This course introduces all 400+ corrective exercises. You will learn what plane each exercise addresses and what misalignment it corrects. It is a self-directed course that is done online, at your own pace.

Symmetry Technician II (Extern) - This course provides an externship in which you will be tested on your knowledge acquired from Level 1. It involves observational hours, either in clinic or live online, and a practical test at the end to certify you as a Symmetry Technician. Once you are certified at this level, you are qualified to use the AlignSmart™ app (Levels 1-2) to access all 400+ corrective exercises.

Symmetry Practitioner I (Intern) - This course is a self-directed online curriculum that teaches you the knowledge behind the AlignSmart Technology™, including how to use the Postural AlignSmart Kit (PAK) to measure, and the basics for creating the patented sequenced routine extracted from the measurements.

Symmetry Practitioner II (Extern) - This course provides an externship in which you will be tested on your knowledge acquired from Level 1. It involves observational hours, either in clinic or live online, and a practical test at the end to certify you as a Symmetry Practitioner. Once you are certified at this level, you are qualified to use the AlignSmart™ app (Level 3) to take clients through a full AlignSmart™ evaluation, creating a unique sequenced routine for each client. This level is designed to add this technology to your existing practice and aid you in your treatment model.

Symmetry Professional Practitioner I (Intern) - This course is a self-directed online curriculum that teaches you the complete knowledge behind the AlignSmart Technology™, including the patented sequencing algorithm for creating the patented sequenced routine extracted from the measurement evaluation.

Symmetry Professional Practitioner II (Extern) - This course provides an externship in which you will be tested on your knowledge acquired from Level 1. It involves observational hours, either in clinic or live online, and a practical test at the end to certify you as a Symmetry Professional Practitioner. Once you are certified at this level, you are qualified to use the AlignSmart™ app (Level 4) to take clients through a full AlignSmart™ evaluation and create a unique

168

sequenced routine for each client. You also have full editing authority. This level includes intensive case study assessments, and full knowledge of how to interact with clients and to use this system as your main treatment model.

Symmetry Whole Business Care I (Intern) - This course is the first of two levels that provide you the opportunity to become a licensed affiliate of Symmetry. It is a self-directed online curriculum that teaches you the complete knowledge behind Symmetry's business operations and processes.

Symmetry Whole Business Care II (Extern) - This course provides an externship in which you will be tested on your knowledge acquired from the first course. It involves observational hours, both in-clinic or live online, and a practical test at the end to certify you as a Symmetry Whole Business Care licensed affiliate. Once you are certified at this level, you are qualified to use the complete Symmetry technology and business systems. This allows you to become a Platinum Affiliate in which your license will give you direct access to our main Symmetry headquarters, with full support and business consultation.

AlignSmart Technology™ for the Practitioner

The following list explains how you as a practitioner can start using our technology, from the free version all the way up to a Level-4 access, which is equivalent to a Symmetry Professional Practitioner. If you are interested in becoming a certified practitioner, visit our certification page on our site and sign up to take one or more Symmetry Technology eCourses (https://symmetryalignsmart.com/certification)

a. **Level 1 Access (Basic):** You can choose from a database of 25 corrective exercises specific for your patient/client based on your own determination. This level is designed for you as a certified or licensed practitioner in your field. The goal is to gain access to a minimal database **without** using our patented evaluation system. This is designed more to aid you in your treatment model based on you evaluating your patient/client. You would not be able to measure, create a report, or generate a routine using our AlignSmart Technology™. But you would be provided a sample of our corrective exercise catalogue to help engage your patient/client in a home-managed program to assist them in your expertise of treatment therapy. If you are a chiropractor, massage therapist, physical therapist, acupuncturist, or personal trainer, for example, this system will be of great use simply to complement your treatments and help patients/clients hold their treatments more permanently.

b. **Level 2 Access (Symmetry Technician I and II):** This level allows you full access to all 400+ exercises in our database. It also formally certifies you as being an expert on understanding and demonstrating these exercises to take your clients/patients through a prescribed and recommended set of exercises. If your current license or certification allows you to already utilize corrective exercises, then you do not need to be certified in our program, but it is recommended. This level also gives you access to our unique messaging system that allows you to privately communicate and support your clients/patients as they experience the corrective exercises you have chosen for them. The emphasis is to hold your clients/patients more accountable with your treatment protocols.

c. **Level 3 Access (Symmetry Practitioner I and II):** This level of certification allows you to use our technology to measure your clients/patients, generate a report, and then create a suggested abbreviated sequence of exercises from a database of over 400+ corrective exercises. You will be certified through our online eCourse, as a Symmetry Practitioner, using our Postural Alignment Kit™ (PAK). You can take the measurements and then train to enter the information into the AlignSmart™ System. The routine that is generated cannot, however, be manipulated or edited, but is derived from our patented algorithm based on you inputting the specific measurements and factors. The routine generated at this level is designed to be conservative, condensed, and non-invasive, but gives you as the practitioner more control in educating and supporting your patient/client using our technology as they perform their routines at home. It is designed, at a higher level, to assist you in your treatment model, but it does not replace your main treatment model. You do, however, need to be certified through our program up to this level to be able to have access. If you want to use the PAK without the use of the app at this level, then that can be a choice as well, or you can have access up to level 3 if you are pre-qualified. Otherwise, if you do want to use the patented system at Level 3 or 4, then you do need to be certified through our online curriculum.

d. **Level 4 Access (Symmetry Professional Practitioner I and II):** This level of certification gives you access to all the previous certifications and to have final editing control over the software. Through this online eCourse, you will understand the entire AlignSmart™ process. Based on the extensive knowledge you possess of your client, you can fine-tune any routine as needed, which gives you ultimate control over your clients/patients' well-being. This level is designed to implement AlignSmart Technology™ as your main treatment program, where we teach you how to use our technology as a primary model and platform for a successful home-managed system. The main emphasis of this level is to make sure the client is a proactive participant in their healing and health process, holding them accountable for the home treatment you determine for them. All other treatments become the tools to aid this process.

Once a practitioner is certified at Level 4, the process of Postural Alignment Technology™ is implemented in the following phases of care. This is our model at Symmetry:

a. **Corrective Phase:** This is called the Postural Detoxification phase. It consists of six sessions scheduled out every other week. In each session your clients/patients will be measured and given a new routine based on the changes made from the previous routine. The client/patient is encouraged to perform each routine twice per day. First to start the day more aligned (assuming the day will pull them out of alignment due to their job or lifestyle), and at the end of the day to correct it again. This encompasses 180 (three months at two times per day) opportunities for a client/patient to perform their specific sequenced routines. We actually educate them to view each routine performance as a treatment session. They are just taking their treatment home with them. Our goal in this phase is to correct a client's/patient's posture from their starting score down to the low 20s or teens. Once they reach this level, not only should they be standing more aligned, but they should also be feeling a lot better. They are now ready for Phase two.

b. **Strength Phase:** This phase is three months and averages every three weeks for each session. The emphasis of the phase is to stabilize the corrections made in the first phase. Each session, the client/patient gets remeasured, taken through a strength routine, and then after one week, they rotate daily with this routine and an earlier corrective routine for two weeks until the next session.

c. **Maintenance Phase:** This phase is where the habit is engrained. Each session occurs once a month. The client is given a new routine at each session and after one week, two earlier routines are mixed in and rotated daily for three weeks until the next session. This phase is focused on teaching a client/patient to understand that when they are on their own, the expectation is that variety is the spice of life, and that consistency is still required to keep them aligned and out of pain.

In my first 15 years of business, my emphasis was only on pain relief, and after three months, clients would get better, then go on their own, and eventually stop doing their routines, because life got in the way. This was the norm until their pain came back. I would inevitably get a phone call explaining their symptoms were returning, and I would ask them what routines they were doing. The answer usually was either that they had stopped doing their routines, or they were only doing one specific routine they liked the best. This is the problem with most clinical therapies. Because pain relief is the main emphasis, once it is gone, people do not think they need to change their habits. I made the same mistake with my own business until I finally realized that I needed to change my own model.

Now, when a new person comes in for the initial consultation, we are very clear that our number one objective if they were to go through our program, is to get their body back to better alignment, stabilize it with strength, then teach them to make it a daily habit, and their pain will dissipate and go away naturally as a result. So, it is not that we do not talk about our clients' pain, we just do not give it as much power as they have been used to with normal treatment programs. When we explain this to a new client, they are left with a decision as to whether they want to make changes in their lives to get out of pain and to stay out of pain. We have a 30-day money-back-guarantee we offer to new clients just in case they are more invested in their pain, and not the long-term solution. This we understand. However, what we also tell our clients is that unless they can take their practitioner home with them every day to be treated, then the chances of that treatment holding is very low, unless it is aided by a program like ours to help complement the treatment.

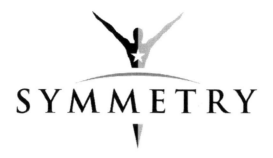

SYMMETRY

GLOSSARY

Active Isometric Exercise- One that provides specific movement of a joint or joints off an isometric holding position and does not displace the body over a measurable distance.

AlignSmart™ system- The patented software system of corrective exercise sequencing.

Anatomical Correctness- When the three planes of the body divide the body equally to form right angles at all eight load bearing joints.

Bipedal- Using only two legs for walking.

Bilateralism- References the fact that our body should be mirror images from side to side.

Center of Mass (COM)- The unique point where the weighted relative position of the distributed mass sums to zero, or true balance (Planes of Motion).

Cerebellum- A small part of our lower brain in the back of the head, plays a vital role in coordinating muscles, controlling many reflexes, and keeping us erect in the earth's gravitational field.

Compensation- The intent to improve any defect by the excessive development or action of another structure or organ of the same structure.

Dynamic Exercise- One that displaces the body over a measurable distance and involve more than one lever.

Dynamic Muscles- Muscles that do change length with external force. Otherwise known as moving muscles.

Egoscue Method- San Diego-based Company who pioneered corrective exercise.

Form follows function- Refers to the time when we develop our structure in the first years, the main intent of our body is to move. Movement during these formative years develops proper form to maintain proper function.

Frontal Plane- Cuts the body into front and back halves. Side-to-side movements.

Fulcrum- The point on which a lever rests or is supported and on which it pivots.

Gravity- A force, which causes any two bodies to be attracted to each other, with the force proportional to the product of their masses and inversely proportional to the square of the distance between them.

Harmonic Tension- In the static standing position, all the muscles, both intrinsic and dynamic, are at their proper length, and therefore leveraged to hold and move the body in its most efficient way possible.

Intrinsic muscles- Muscles that do not change length with external force. Otherwise known as postural muscles.

Isometric Exercise- One that provides **work without movement** and describes most of the Symmetry Postures. These exercises can include more isometric stretching (i.e., Piriformis Crossovers).

Lever- A rigid bar resting on a pivot, used to help move a heavy or rigidly fixed load with one end when pressure is applied to the other (i.e. bones).

Locomotor Unit- Comprised of the pelvis and legs.

Muscle Balance and Function (MBF)- Geoff Gluckman, a disciple of Pete Egoscue, created a deeper layer of understanding of The Egoscue Method.

Negative structural patterns- This refers to how our environment today is not conducive to supporting our frame as it was intended. Automation vs hands-on work.

Newton's Third Law- For every action, there is an equal and opposite reaction.

Passenger Unit- Comprised of the upper torso as it relates to sitting on top of the Locomotor unit.

Passive Exercise- One that has **no work** associated with it. It is typically a releasing exercise or a resting exercise such as the Static Floor.

Physiological Correctness- When the organ systems of the body operate effectively and efficiently.

Planes of Motion- Three physiological planes that describe the range of motion in the body. These planes represent the X, Y, and Z axis in the Cartesian coordinate system.

Plumb Line- a line often used by contractors as a reference to the force of gravity and right angles.

Postural Detoxification- The time it takes to remove old negative compensation patterns.

Postural Red Flags- Anything that is visually skewed from right angles around three-dimensional space.

Pulley- A device for overcoming resistance at one point by applying force at some other point (i.e. muscles).

Righting Reflex- A reflex that corrects the orientation of the body when it is taken out of its normal upright position.

Sagittal Plane- Cuts the body into left and right halves. Forward and backward movements.

Scoliosis (Functional) - Lateral shifting of the spine due to misalignments developed via environmental compensation.

Scoliosis (Structural) - Lateral shifting and rotation of the spine due to a genetic predisposition (born with it).

Segmental Alignment- The parts of the skeleton acting together around the force of gravity.

Severity-Disparity Chart™- The chart that provides the quantifiable values for each measurement to calculate the planar relationships.

Sympathetic Nervous System- The sympathetic nervous system's primary process is to stimulate the body's fight-flight-or-freeze response. It is, however, constantly active at a basic level to maintain homeostasis.

Thoracic Vertebrae- The middle section of the spine, composed of 12 vertebrae.

Transverse Plane- Cuts the body into top and bottom halves. Twisting movements.

Vertical Loadbearing- A body vertically erect around the force of gravity with full weight intensity distributed throughout the loadbearing joints.

Vestibular System- A sensory system that is responsible for providing our brain with information about motion, head position, and spatial orientation.

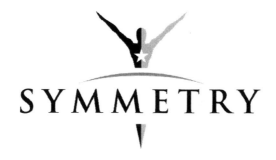

BIBLIOGRAPHY

Commercial Aspects (n.d., 2019)
https://breakingmuscle.com/fitness/the-future-of-fitness-who-will-win-the-gym-wars

Gluckman, G. (1998). Muscle Balance and Function Development (MBF system) Training Manual. San Diego: Dynamics of Physical Development Consultants.

Isometric Training:
https://breakingmuscle.com/fitness/isometric-training-what-it-is-and-how-to-do-it-correctly

National Institute of Health:
www.ninds.nih.gov/Disorders/All-Disorders/Back-Pain-Information-Page

Naturally Lower Your Blood Pressure:
https://draxe.com/natural-ways-to-lower-blood-pressure/

Natural Remedy for Depression:
https://draxe.com/natural-remedies-depression/

Science Daily, Journal of Pain:
https://www.sciencedaily.com/releases/2012/09/1209110
91100.htm

National Bureau of Economic Research; Valuing Pain Using the Subjective Well-Being Method; Working Paper 23649: http://www.nber.org/papers/w23649

Napier, J. (1967). The Antiquity of Human Walking. In Scientific American (Ed.), Human Variation and Origins: An Introduction to Human Biology and Evaluation (pp. 116-126). San Francisco: W. H. Freeman.

Perry, J. (1992). Gait Analysis: Normal and Pathological Function. New York: McGraw-Hill.

Todd, M. E. (1937). The Thinking Body. New York: Hoeber.

Vernikos, Joan Ph.D. Sitting Kills, Moving Heals.